SEVENTH EDITION

RESPIRATORY
PHYSIOLOGY

THE ESSENTIALS

SEVENTH EDITION

RESPIRATORY PHYSIOLOGY

THE ESSENTIALS

JOHN B. WEST, M.D., Ph.D., D.Sc.

Professor of Medicine and Physiology
University of California, San Diego
School of Medicine
La Jolla, California

LIPPINCOTT WILLIAMS & WILKINS
A **Wolters Kluwer** Company
Philadelphia • Baltimore • New York • London
Buenos Aires • Hong Kong • Sydney • Tokyo

Editor: Betty Sun
Managing Editor: Crystal Taylor
Marketing Manager: Joe Schott
Production Editor: Jennifer Glazer
Compositor: Maryland Composition
Printer: R. R. Donnelley

351 West Camden Street
Baltimore, Maryland 21201-2436 USA

530 Walnut Street
Philadelphia, Pennsylvania 19106-3621 USA

The publisher is not responsible (as a matter of product liability, negligence, or otherwise) for
any injury resulting from any material contained herein. This publication contains information
relating to general principles of medical care which should not be construed as specific instruc-
tions for individual patients. Manufacturers' product information and package inserts should be
reviewed for current information, including contraindications, dosages and precautions.

Printed in the United States of America

First Edition, 1974
Second Edition, 1979
Third Edition, 1985
Fourth Edition, 1990
Fifth Edition, 1995
Sixth Edition, 2000

French translation, 1975, 1986; Spanish translation, 1976; Iranian translation, 1976; Portuguese
translation, 1977; Italian translation, 1978; Chinese translation, 1979; Japanese translation,
1981; Dutch translation, 1981; Turkish translation, 1982; Bahasa Malaysia translation, 1984;
Russian translation, 1988; Greek translation,1988; Indonesian translation, 1990; French trans-
lation, 1995; Greek translation, 1995; Spanish translation, 1996; Japanese translation, 1997.

Library of Congress Cataloging-in-Publication Data

West, John B. (John Burnard)
    Respiratory physiology : the essentials / John B. West.—7th ed.
        p. ; cm.
    Includes bibliographical references and index.
    ISBN-13: 978-0-7817-5152-0
    ISBN 0-7817-5152-7
        1. Respiration I. Title.
    [DNLM: 1. Respiratory Physiology. WF 102 W518r 2004]
    QP121.W43 2004
    612.2—dc22

                                                            2004044149

*The publishers have made every effort to trace the copyright holders for borrowed material. If they have
inadvertently overlooked any, they will be pleased to make the necessary arrangements at the first op-
portunity.*

To purchase additional copies of this book, call our customer service department at **(800) 638-
3030** or fax orders to **(301) 824-7390.** International customers should call **(301) 714-2324.**

Visit Lippincott Williams & Wilkins on the Internet: http://www.lww.com.

06 07 08
4 5 6 7 8 9 10

To P.H.W.

Preface

This book first appeared 30 years ago, and it has been well received and translated into 13 languages. It is appropriate to briefly review the objectives.

First, the book is intended as an introductory text for medical students and allied health students. As such, it will normally be used in conjunction with a course of lectures, and this is the case at University of California, San Diego (UCSD) School of Medicine. Indeed, the first edition was written because I believed that there was no appropriate textbook at that time to accompany the first year physiology course.

Second, the book is written as a review for residents and fellows in such areas as pulmonary medicine, anesthesiology, and internal medicine, particularly to help them prepare for licensing and other examinations. Here the requirements are somewhat different. The reader is familiar with the general area but needs to have his or her memory jogged on various points, and the many didactic diagrams are particularly important.

It might be useful to add a word or two about how the book meshes with the lectures to the first year medical students at UCSD. We are limited to about twelve 50-minute lectures on respiratory physiology supplemented by two laboratories and three discussion groups. The lectures follow the individual chapters of the book closely, with most chapters corresponding to a single lecture. The exceptions are that Chapter 5 has two lectures (one on normal gas exchange, hypoventilation, and shunt; another on the difficult topic of ventilation-perfusion relationships); Chapter 6 has two lectures (one on blood-gas transport and another on acid-base balance); Chapter 7 has two lectures (on statics and dynamics), and if the schedule of the course allows, the section on polluted atmospheres in Chapter 9 is expanded to include an additional lecture on defense systems of the lung. There is no lecture on Chapter 10 "Tests of Pulmonary Function" because this is not part of the core course. It is included partly for interest and partly because of its importance to people who work in pulmonary function laboratories.

Several colleagues have suggested that Chapter 6 on gas transport should come earlier in the book because knowledge of the oxygen dissociation curve is needed to properly understand diffusion across the blood-gas barrier. In fact, we make this switch in our lecture course. However, the various chapters of the book can stand alone, and I prefer the present ordering of chapters because it leads to a nice flow of ideas as the cartoons at the beginning of each chapter indicate. The order of chapters also probably makes it easier for the reader who is reviewing material.

It is sometimes argued that Chapter 7 "Mechanics of Breathing" should come earlier, for example, with Chapter 2 "Ventilation." My experience of over 35 years of teaching is strongly against this. The topic of mechanics is so complex and difficult for the present-day medical student that it is best dealt with separately, and later in the course when the students are more prepared for the concepts. Parenthetically, it seems that many modern medical students find concepts of pressure, flow, and resistance much more difficult than was the case 25 years ago, whereas, of course, they breeze through any discussion of molecular biology.

Some colleagues have recommended that more space should be devoted to sample calculations using the equations in the text and various clinical examples. My belief is that these topics are well-suited to the lectures, which can then embellish the basic information. Indeed, if the calculations and clinical examples were included in the book, there would be precious little to talk about. Many of the questions at the end of each chapter require calculations.

The present edition has been thoroughly updated including changes in the sections on structure and function, hypoxic pulmonary vasoconstriction, gas transport by the blood, relaxation pressure-volume curve, dynamic compression of the airways, lung receptors, and perinatal respiration. Several of the diagrams have been improved. Extensive changes in the format have been made to help the reader. These include summaries at the beginning of each chapter. In addition the questions have now been recast in the USMLE format and they have been placed at the end of each chapter.

Heroic efforts have been made to keep the book lean, in spite of enormous temptations to fatten it. Occasionally, medical students wonder if the book is too superficial. I disagree; in fact, if pulmonary fellows beginning their training in intensive care units fully understood all the material on gas exchange and mechanics, the world would be a better place.

Many students and teachers have written to query statements in the book or to make suggestions for improvement. I respond personally to every point that is raised and much appreciate this input.

Contents

1

Structure and Function
How the Architecture of the Lung Subserves Its Function

Blood-Gas Interface	**Stability of Alveoli**
Airways and Airflow	**Removal of Inhaled Particles**
Blood Vessels and Flow	

We begin with a short review of the relationships between structure and function in the lung. First we look at blood-gas interface where the exchange of the respiratory gases occurs. Next we look at how oxygen is brought to the interface through the airways, and then how the blood removes the oxygen from the lung. Finally two potential problems of the lung are briefly addressed: how the alveoli maintain their stability, and how the lung is kept clean in a polluted environment.

The lung is for gas exchange. Its prime function is to allow oxygen to move from the air into the venous blood and carbon dioxide to move out. The lung does other jobs too. It metabolizes some compounds, filters unwanted materials from the circulation, and acts as a reservoir for blood. But its cardinal function is to exchange gas, and we shall therefore begin at the blood-gas interface where the gas exchange occurs.

1

Blood-Gas Interface

Oxygen and carbon dioxide move between air and blood by simple diffusion, that is, from an area of high to low partial pressure,* much as water runs downhill. Fick's law of diffusion states that the amount of gas that moves across a sheet of tissue is proportional to the area of the sheet but inversely proportional to its thickness. The blood-gas barrier is exceedingly thin (Figure 1-1) and has an area of between 50 and 100 square meters. It is therefore well suited to its function of gas exchange.

How is it possible to obtain such a prodigious surface area for diffusion inside the limited thoracic cavity? This is done by wrapping the small blood vessels (capillaries) around an enormous number of small air sacs called *alveoli* (Figure 1-2). There are about 300 million alveoli in the human lung, each about 1/3 mm in diameter. If they were spheres,[†] their total surface area would be 85 square meters, but their volume only 4 liters. By contrast, a single sphere of this volume would have an internal surface area of only 1/100 square meter. Thus, the lung generates this large diffusion area by being divided into myriad units.

Gas is brought to one side of the blood-gas interface by *airways*, and blood to the other side by *blood vessels*.

Airways and Airflow

The airways consist of a series of branching tubes which become narrower, shorter, and more numerous as they penetrate deeper into the lung (Figure 1-3). The *trachea* divides into right and left main bronchi, which in turn divide into lobar, then segmental bronchi. This process continues down to the *terminal bronchioles*, which are the smallest airways without alveoli. All of these bronchi make up the *conducting airways*. Their function is to lead inspired air to the gas exchanging regions of the lung (Figure 1-4). Because the conducting airways contain no alveoli and therefore take no part in gas exchange, they constitute the *anatomic dead space*. Its volume is about 150 ml.

The terminal bronchioles divide into *respiratory bronchioles*, which have occasional alveoli budding from their walls. Finally, we come to the *alveolar ducts*, which are completely lined with alveoli. This alveolated region of the lung where the gas exchange occurs is known as the *respiratory zone*. The portion of lung dis-

---

* The partial pressure of a gas is found by multiplying its concentration by the total pressure. For example, dry air has 20.93% O_2. Its partial pressure (P_{O_2}) at sea level (barometric pressure 760 mm Hg) is $20.93/100 \times 760 = 159$ mm Hg. When air is inhaled into the upper airways, it is warmed and moistened, and the water vapor pressure is then 47 mm Hg, so that the total dry gas pressure is only $760 - 47 = 713$ mm Hg. The P_{O_2} of inspired air is therefore $20.93/100 \times 713 = 149$ mm Hg. A liquid exposed to a gas until equilibration takes place has the same partial pressure as the gas. For a more complete description of the gas laws, see Appendix A.

[†] The alveoli are not spherical but polyhedral. Nor is the whole of their surface available for diffusion (see Figure 1-1). These numbers are therefore only approximate.

Figure 1-1. Electron micrograph showing a pulmonary capillary (C) in the alveolar wall. Note the extremely thin blood-gas barrier of about 0.3 μm in some places. The *large arrow* indicates the diffusion path from alveolar gas to the interior of the erythrocyte (EC) and includes the layer of surfactant (not shown in the preparation), alveolar epithelium (EP), interstitium (IN), capillary endothelium (EN), and plasma. Parts of structural cells called fibroblasts (FB), basement membrane (BM), and a nucleus of an endothelial cell are also seen.

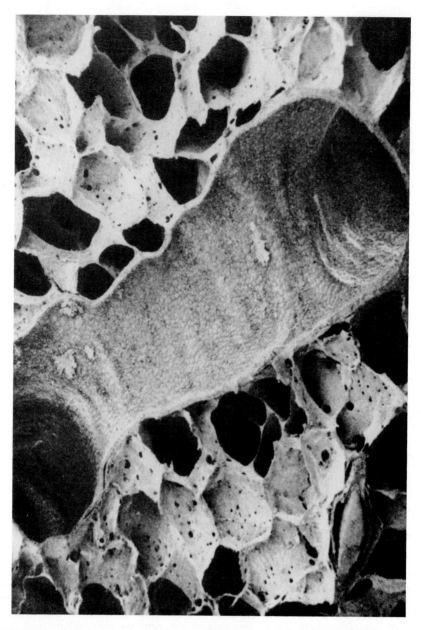

Figure 1-2. Section of lung showing many alveoli and a small bronchiole. The pulmonary capillaries run in the walls of the alveoli (Figure 1-1). The holes in the alveolar walls are the pores of Kohn.

Figure 1-3. Cast of the airways of a human lung. The alveoli have been pruned away, allowing the conducting airways from the trachea to the terminal bronchioles to be seen.

tal to a terminal bronchiole forms an anatomical unit called the *acinus*. The distance from the terminal bronchiole to the most distal alveolus is only a few mm, but the respiratory zone makes up most of the lung, its volume being about 2.5 to 3 liters during rest.

During inspiration, the volume of the thoracic cavity increases and air is drawn into the lung. The increase in volume is brought about partly by contraction of the diaphragm, which causes it to descend, and partly by the action of the intercostal muscles, which raise the ribs, thus increasing the cross-sectional area of the thorax. Inspired air flows down to about the terminal bronchioles by bulk flow, like water through a hose. Beyond that point, the combined cross-sectional

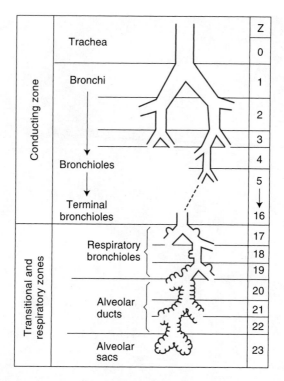

Figure 1-4. Idealization of the human airways according to Weibel. Note that the first 16 generations (Z) make up the conducting airways, and the last 7, the respiratory zone (or the transitional and respiratory zone).

area of the airways is so enormous because of the large number of branches (Figure 1-5) that the forward velocity of the gas becomes small. Diffusion of gas within the airways then takes over as the dominant mechanism of ventilation in the respiratory zone. The rate of diffusion of gas molecules within the airways is so rapid and the distances to be covered so short that differences in concentration within the acinus are virtually abolished within a second. However, because the velocity of gas falls rapidly in the region of the terminal bronchioles, inhaled dust frequently settles out there.

Airways

- Divided into a conducting zone and a respiratory zone
- Volume of the anatomic dead space is about 150 ml
- Volume of the alveolar region is about 2.5–3.0 liters
- Gas movement in the alveolar region is chiefly by diffusion

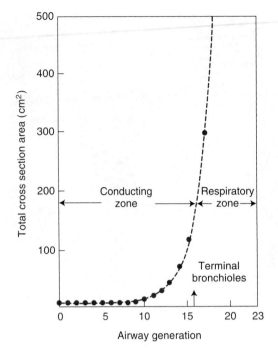

Figure 1-5. Diagram to show the extremely rapid increase in total cross-sectional area of the airways in the respiratory zone (compare Figure 1-4). As a result, the forward velocity of the gas during inspiration becomes very small in the region of the respiratory bronchioles, and gaseous diffusion becomes the chief mode of ventilation.

The lung is elastic and returns passively to its preinspiratory volume during resting breathing. It is remarkably easy to distend. A normal breath of about 500 ml, for example, requires a distending pressure of less than 3 cm water. By contrast, a child's balloon may need a pressure of 30 cm water for the same change in volume.

The pressure required to move gas through the airways is also very small. During normal inspiration, an air flow rate of 1 liter/sec requires a pressure drop along the airways of less than 2 cm water. Compare a smoker's pipe which needs a pressure of about 500 cm water for the same flow rate.

Blood Vessels and Flow

The pulmonary blood vessels also form a series of branching tubes from the *pulmonary artery* to the *capillaries* and back to the *pulmonary veins*. Initially, the arteries, veins, and bronchi run close together, but toward the periphery of the lung, the veins move away to pass between the lobules, whereas the arteries and bronchi travel together down the centers of the lobules. The capillaries form a dense network in the walls of the alveoli (Figure 1-6). The diameter of a capillary

500μ

Figure 1-6. View of an alveolar wall (in the frog) showing the dense network of capillaries. A small artery (*left*) and vein (*right*) can also be seen. The individual capillary segments are so short that the blood forms an almost continuous sheet.

segment is about 10 μm, just large enough for a red blood cell. The lengths of the segments are so short that the dense network forms an almost continuous sheet of blood in the alveolar wall, a very efficient arrangement for gas exchange. Alveolar walls are not often seen face on, as in Figure 1-6. The usual, thin microscopic cross section (Figure 1-7) shows the red blood cells in the capillaries and emphasizes the enormous exposure of blood to alveolar gas, with only the thin blood-gas barrier intervening (compare Figure 1-1).

The extreme thinness of the blood-gas barrier means that the capillaries are easily damaged. Increasing the pressure in the capillaries to high levels or inflating the lung to high volumes, for example, can raise the wall stresses of the capillaries to the point at which ultrastructural changes can occur. The capillaries then leak plasma and even red blood cells into the alveolar spaces.

The pulmonary artery receives the whole output of the right heart, but the resistance of the pulmonary circuit is astonishingly small. A mean pulmonary arterial pressure of only about 20 cm water (about 15 mm Hg) is required for a flow of 6 liters/min (the same flow through a soda straw needs 120 cm water).

Each red blood cell spends about 3/4 sec in the capillary network and during this time probably traverses two or three alveoli. So efficient is the anatomy for

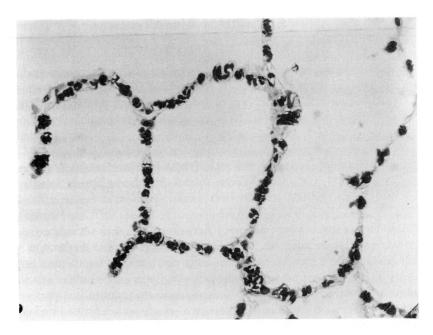

Figure 1-7. Microscopic section of dog lung showing capillaries in the alveolar walls. The blood-gas barrier is so thin that it cannot be identified here (compare Figure 1-1). This section was prepared from lung that was rapidly frozen while being perfused.

gas exchange that this brief time is sufficient for virtually complete equilibration of oxygen and carbon dioxide between alveolar gas and capillary blood.

The lung has an additional blood system, the bronchial circulation, which supplies the conducting airways down to about the terminal bronchioles. Some of this blood is carried away from the lung via the pulmonary veins and some enters the systemic circulation. The flow through the bronchial circulation is a mere fraction of that through the pulmonary circulation, and the lung can function fairly well without it, for example, following lung transplantation.

To conclude this brief account of the functional anatomy of the lung, let us glance at two special problems that the lung has overcome.

Blood Vessels

- Whole of the output of the right heart goes to the lung
- Diameter of the capillaries is about 10 μm
- Thickness of much of the blood-gas barrier is less than 0.3 μm
- Blood spends about 3/4 sec in the capillaries

Stability of Alveoli

The lung can be regarded as a collection of 300 million bubbles, each 0.3 mm in diameter. Such a structure is inherently unstable. Because of the surface tension of the liquid lining the alveoli, relatively large forces develop that tend to collapse alveoli. Fortunately, some of the cells lining the alveoli secrete a material called *surfactant*, which dramatically lowers the surface tension of the alveolar lining layer (see Chapter 7). As a consequence, the stability of the alveoli is enormously increased, although collapse of small air spaces is always a potential problem and frequently occurs in disease.

Removal of Inhaled Particles

With its surface area of 50 to100 square meters, the lung presents the largest surface of the body to an increasingly hostile environment. Various mechanisms for dealing with inhaled particles have been developed (see Chapter 9). Large particles are filtered out in the nose. Smaller particles that deposit in the conducting airways are removed by a moving staircase of mucus that continually sweeps debris up to the epiglottis, where it is swallowed. The mucus, secreted by mucous glands and also by goblet cells in the bronchial walls, is propelled by millions of tiny cilia, which move rhythmically under normal conditions but are paralyzed by some inhaled toxins.

The alveoli have no cilia, and particles that deposit there are engulfed by large wandering cells called macrophages. The foreign material is then removed from the lung via the lymphatics or the blood flow. Blood cells such as leukocytes also participate in the defense reaction to foreign material.

QUESTIONS

For each question, choose the one best answer.

1. Which of the following statements about the blood-gas barrier of the human lung is **FALSE**?
   A. Much of the blood-gas barrier has a thickness of less than 0.3 μm.
   B. The total area of the blood-gas barrier exceeds 50 square meters.
   C. Most of the area of the alveolar wall is occupied by capillaries.
   D. If the pressure in the capillaries rises to unphysiologically high levels, the blood-gas barrier can be damaged.
   E. Oxygen crosses the blood-gas barrier by active transport.
2. When oxygen moves through the thin side of the blood-gas barrier from the alveolar gas to the hemoglobin of the red blood cell it traverses the following layers in order:
   A. Epithelial cell, surfactant, interstitium, endothelial cell, plasma, red cell membrane.
   B. Surfactant, epithelial cell, interstitium, endothelial cell, plasma, red cell membrane.

C. Surfactant, endothelial cell, interstitium, epithelial cell, plasma, red cell membrane.

D. Epithelium, interstitium, endothelial cell, plasma, red cell membrane.

E. Surfactant, epithelial cell, interstitium, endothelial cell, red cell membrane.

3. What is the Po_2 (in mm Hg) of moist inspired gas of a climber on the summit of Mt. Everest (assume barometric pressure is 247 mm Hg)?
   A. 32
   B. 42
   C. 52
   D. 62
   E. 72

4. Which of the following statements about the airways of the human lung is **FALSE**?
   A. The volume of the conducting zone is about 150 ml.
   B. The volume of the rest of the lung during resting conditions is about 2.5–3.0 liters.
   C. A respiratory bronchiole can be distinguished from a terminal bronchiole because the former has alveoli in its walls.
   D. On the average there are about 3 branchings of the conducting airways before the first alveoli appear in their walls.
   E. In the respiratory bronchioles the predominant mode of gas flow is diffusion rather than convection.

5. Which of the following statements about the blood vessels of the human lung is **FALSE**?
   A. The pulmonary arteries form a branching pattern which matches that of the airways.
   B. The average diameter of the capillaries is about 50 μm.
   C. Most of the surface of the alveoli is covered with capillaries.
   D. On the average blood spends about 3/4 sec in the capillaries.
   E. The mean pressure in the pulmonary artery is only about 15 mm Hg at rest.

6. Which of the following statements about the removal of inhaled dust in the lung is **FALSE**?
   A. Very small particles are filtered out by the nose.
   B. Particles that deposit on the airways are removed by the mucus escalator.
   C. The escalator is propelled by millions of tiny cilia.
   D. The mucus comes from mucous glands and goblet cells in the bronchial walls.
   E. Particles that reach the alveoli are engulfed by macrophages.

2

Ventilation
How Gas Gets to the Alveoli

We now look in more detail at how oxygen is brought to the blood-gas barrier by the process of ventilation. First lung volumes are briefly reviewed. Then total ventilation and alveolar ventilation, that is the amount of fresh gas getting to the alveoli, are discussed. The lung that does not participate in gas exchange is dealt with under anatomic and physiologic dead space. Finally the uneven distribution of ventilation caused by gravity is introduced.

The next three chapters concern how inspired air gets to the alveoli, how gases cross the blood-gas interface, and how they are removed from the lung by the blood. These functions are carried out by ventilation, diffusion, and blood flow, respectively.

Figure 2-1 is a highly simplified diagram of a lung. The various bronchi that make up the conducting airways (Figures 1-3 and 1-4) are now represented by a single tube labeled anatomic dead space. This leads into the gas-exchanging region of the lung, which is bounded by the blood-gas interface and the pulmonary capillary blood. With each inspiration, about 500 ml of air enter the lung (*tidal volume*). Note how small a proportion of the total lung volume is represented by

13

VOLUMES   FLOWS

Figure 2-1. Diagram of a lung showing typical volumes and flows. There is considerable variation around these values.

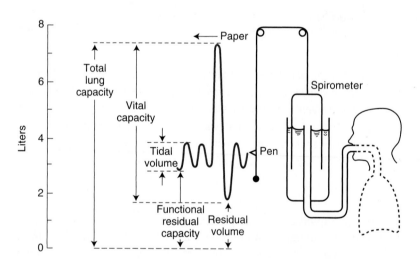

Figure 2-2. Lung volumes. Note that the total lung capacity, functional residual capacity, and residual volume cannot be measured with the spirometer.

the anatomic dead space. Also note the very small volume of capillary blood compared with that of alveolar gas (compare Figure 1-7).

Lung Volumes

Before looking at the movement of gas into the lung, a brief glance at the static volumes of the lung is helpful. Some of these can be measured with a spirometer (Figure 2-2). During exhalation, the bell goes up and the pen down, marking a moving chart. First, normal breathing can be seen (*tidal volume*). Next the subject took a maximal inspiration and followed this by a maximal expiration. The exhaled volume is called the *vital capacity*. However, some gas remained in the lung after a maximal expiration; this is the *residual volume*. The volume of gas in the lung after a normal expiration is the *functional residual capacity*.

Neither the functional residual capacity nor the residual volume can be measured with a simple spirometer. However, a gas dilution technique can be used as shown in Figure 2-3. The subject is connected to a spirometer containing a known concentration of helium, which is virtually insoluble in blood. After some breaths, the helium concentrations in the spirometer and lung become the same.

Because no helium has been lost, the amount of helium present before equilibration (concentration times volume) is:

$$C_1 \times V_1$$

and equals the amount after equilibration:

$$C_2 \times (V_1 + V_2)$$

From this:

$$V_2 = V_1 (C_1 - C_2) / C_2$$

Before equilibration   **After equilibration**

$$C_1 \times V_1 = C_2 \times (V_1 + V_2)$$

Figure 2-3. Measurement of the functional residual capacity by helium dilution.

Figure 2-4. Measurement of functional residual capacity (FRC) with a body plethysmograph. When the subject makes an inspiratory effort against a closed airway, he slightly increases the volume of his lung, airway pressure decreases, and box pressure increases. From Boyle's law, lung volume is obtained (see text).

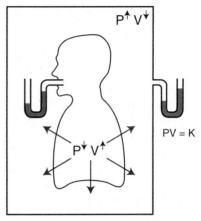

In practice, oxygen is added to the spirometer during equilibration to make up for that consumed by the subject, and also carbon dioxide is absorbed.

Another way of measuring the functional residual capacity (FRC) is with a body plethysmograph (Figure 2-4). This is a large airtight box, like an old telephone booth, in which the subject sits. At the end of a normal expiration, a shutter closes the mouthpiece and the subject is asked to make respiratory efforts. As the subject tries to inhale, he (or she) expands the gas in his lungs, and lung volume increases, and the box pressure rises because its gas volume decreases. Boyle's law states that pressure × volume is constant (at constant temperature).

Therefore, if the pressures in the box before and after the inspiratory effort are P_1 and P_2, respectively, V_1 is the pre-inspiratory box volume and ΔV is the change in volume of the box (or lung), we can write:

$$P_1 V_1 = P_2 (V_1 - \Delta V)$$

Thus ΔV can be obtained.

Next, Boyle's Law is applied to the gas in the lung. Now:

$$P_3 V_2 = P_4 (V_2 + \Delta V)$$

where P_3 and P_4 are the mouth pressures before and after the inspiratory effort, and V_2 is the FRC. Thus FRC can be obtained.

The body plethysmograph measures the total volume of gas in the lung, including any that is trapped behind closed airways (an example is shown in Figure 7-9) and that therefore does not communicate with the mouth. By contrast, the helium dilution method measures only communicating gas, or ventilated lung volume. In young normal subjects, these volumes are virtually the same, but in patients with lung disease, the ventilated volume may be considerably less than the total volume because of gas trapped behind obstructed airways.

Lung Volumes

- Tidal volume and vital capacity can be measured with a simple spirometer
- Total lung capacity, functional residual capacity and residual volume need an additional measurement by helium dilution or the body plethysmograph
- Helium is used because of its very low solubility in blood
- The body plethysmograph depends on Boyle's Law PV=K at constant temperature

---

Ventilation

Suppose the volume exhaled with each breath is 500 ml (Figure 2-1) and there are 15 breaths/min. Then the total volume leaving the lung each minute is 500 $\times$ 15 = 7500 ml/min. This is known as the *total ventilation*. The volume of air entering the lung is very slightly greater because more oxygen is taken in than carbon dioxide is given out.

However, not all the air that passes the lips reaches the alveolar gas compartment where gas exchange occurs. Of each 500 ml inhaled in Figure 2-1, 150 ml remain behind in the anatomic dead space. Thus, the volume of fresh gas entering the respiratory zone each minute is (500 − 150) $\times$ 15 or 5250 ml/min. This is called the *alveolar ventilation* and is of key importance because it represents the amount of fresh inspired air available for gas exchange (strictly, the alveolar ventilation is also measured on expiration, but the volume is almost the same.)

The total ventilation can be measured easily by having the subject breathe through a valve box that separates the inspired from the expired gas, and collecting all the expired gas in a bag. The alveolar ventilation is more difficult to determine. One way is to measure the volume of the anatomic dead space (see below) and calculate the dead space ventilation (volume $\times$ respiratory frequency). This is then subtracted from the total ventilation.

We can summarize this conveniently with symbols (Figure 2-5). Using V to denote volume, and the subscripts T, D, and A to denote tidal, dead space, and alveolar, respectively:

$$V_T = V_D + V_A{}^*$$

therefore, $\qquad\qquad V_T \cdot n = V_D \cdot n + V_A \cdot n$

where n is the respiratory frequency.

Therefore, $\qquad\qquad\qquad \dot{V}_E = \dot{V}_D + \dot{V}_A$

where $\dot{V}$ means volume per unit time, $\dot{V}_E$ is expired total ventilation, and $\dot{V}_D$ and $\dot{V}_A$ are the dead space and alveolar ventilations, respectively (see Appendix A for a summary of symbols).

---

*Note that V_A here means the volume of alveolar gas in the tidal volume, not the total volume of alveolar gas in the lung.

Thus,

$$\dot{V}_A = \dot{V}_E - \dot{V}_D$$

A difficulty with this method is that the anatomic dead space is not easy to measure, although a value for it can be assumed with little error. Note that alveolar ventilation can be increased by raising either tidal volume or respiratory frequency (or both). Increasing tidal volume is often more effective because this reduces the proportion of each breath occupied by the anatomic dead space.

Another way of measuring alveolar ventilation in normal subjects is from the concentration of CO_2 in expired gas (Figure 2-5). Because no gas exchange occurs in the anatomic dead space, there is no CO_2 there at the end of inspiration (we can neglect the small amount of CO_2 in the air.) Thus, because all the expired CO_2 comes from the alveolar gas,

$$\dot{V}_{CO_2} = \dot{V}_A \times \frac{\% \ CO_2}{100}$$

where $\dot{V}_{CO_2}$ means the volume of CO_2 exhaled per unit time.

Rearranging, $$\dot{V}_A = \frac{\dot{V}_{CO_2} \times 100}{\% \ CO_2}$$

The $\% \ CO_2/100$ is often called the fractional concentration and is denoted by F_{CO_2}. Thus, the alveolar ventilation can be obtained by dividing the CO_2 output by the alveolar fractional concentration of this gas.

Note that the partial pressure of CO_2 (denoted P_{CO_2}) is proportional to the fractional concentration of the gas in the alveoli, or $P_{CO_2} = F_{CO_2} \times K$ where K is a constant.

Therefore, $$\dot{V}_A = \frac{\dot{V}_{CO_2}}{P_{CO_2}} \times K$$

Figure 2-5. The tidal volume (V_T) is a mixture of gas from the anatomic dead space (V_D) and a contribution from the alveolar gas (V_A). The concentrations of CO_2 are shown by the *dots*. F, fractional concentration; I, inspired; E, expired. Compare Figure 1-4.

Because in normal subjects the P_{CO_2} of alveolar gas and arterial blood are virtually identical, the arterial P_{CO_2} can be used to determine alveolar ventilation. The relation between alveolar ventilation and P_{CO_2} is of crucial importance. If the alveolar ventilation is halved (and CO_2 production remains unchanged), for example, the alveolar and arterial P_{CO_2} will double.

Anatomic Dead Space

This is the volume of the conducting airways (Figures 1-3 and 1-4). The normal value is about 150 ml, and it increases with large inspirations because of the traction or pull exerted on the bronchi by the surrounding lung parenchyma. The dead space also depends on the size and posture of the subject.

The volume of the anatomic dead space can be measured by *Fowler's method*. The subject breathes through a valve box, and the sampling tube of a rapid nitrogen analyzer continuously samples gas at the lips (Figure 2-6A). Following a single inspiration of 100% O_2, the N_2 concentration rises as the dead space gas is increasingly washed out by alveolar gas. Finally, an almost uniform gas concentration is seen representing pure alveolar gas. This phase is often called the alveolar "plateau," although in normal subjects it is not quite flat, and in patients with lung disease it may rise steeply. Expired volume is also recorded.

The dead space is found by plotting N_2 concentration against expired volume and drawing a vertical line such that area A is equal to area B in Figure 2-6B. The dead space is the volume expired up to the vertical line. In effect, this method measures the volume of the conducting airways down to the midpoint of the transition from dead space to alveolar gas.

Physiologic Dead Space

Another way of measuring dead space is *Bohr's method*. Figure 2-5 shows that all the expired CO_2 comes from the alveolar gas and none from the dead space. Therefore, we can write

$$V_T \cdot F_E = V_A \cdot F_A$$

now,

$$V_T = V_A + V_D$$

therefore,

$$V_A = V_T - V_D$$

substituting

$$V_T \cdot F_E = (V_T - V_D) \cdot F_A$$

whence

$$\frac{V_D}{V_T} = \frac{F_A - F_E}{F_A}$$

We saw earlier that the partial pressure of a gas is proportional to its concentration. Thus,

$$\frac{V_D}{V_T} = \frac{P_{A_{CO_2}} - P_{E_{CO_2}}}{P_{A_{CO_2}}} \quad \text{(Bohr equation)}$$

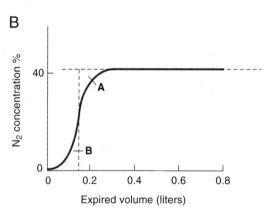

Figure 2-6. Fowler's method of measuring the anatomic dead space with a rapid N_2 analyzer. **A** shows that following a test inspiration of 100% O_2, the N_2 concentration rises during expiration to an almost level "plateau" representing pure alveolar gas. In **B**, N_2 concentration is plotted against expired volume, and the dead space is the volume up to the *vertical dashed line*, which makes the areas *A* and *B* equal.

where A and E refer to alveolar and mixed expired, respectively (see Appendix A). The normal ratio of dead space to tidal volume is in the range 0.2 to 0.35 during resting breathing. In normal subjects, the P_{CO_2} in alveolar gas and that in arterial blood are virtually identical so that the equation is therefore often written

$$\frac{V_D}{V_T} = \frac{Pa_{CO_2} - PE_{CO_2}}{Pa_{CO_2}}$$

Ventilation

- Total ventilation is tidal volume × respiratory frequency
- Alveolar ventilation is the amount of fresh gas getting to the alveoli, or $(V_T - V_D) \times n$
- Anatomic dead space is the volume of the conducting airways, about 150 ml
- Physiologic dead space is the volume of gas that does not eliminate CO_2
- The two dead spaces are almost the same in normal subjects, but the physiologic dead space is increased in many lung diseases

---

It should be noted that Fowler's and Bohr's methods measure somewhat different things. Fowler's method measures the volume of the conducting airways down to the level where the rapid dilution of inspired gas occurs with gas already in the lung. This volume is determined by the geometry of the rapidly expanding airways (Figure 1-5), and because it reflects the morphology of the lung, it is called the *anatomic dead space*. Bohr's method measures the volume of the lung that does not eliminate CO_2. Because this is a functional measurement, the volume is called the *physiologic dead space*. In normal subjects, the volumes are very nearly the same. However, in patients with lung disease, the physiologic dead space may be considerably larger because of inequality of blood flow and ventilation within the lung (see Chapter 5).

Regional Differences of Ventilation

So far we have been assuming that all regions of the normal lung have the same ventilation. However, it has been shown that the lower regions of the lung ventilate better than do the upper zones. This can be demonstrated if a subject inhales radioactive xenon gas (Figure 2-7). When the xenon-133 enters the

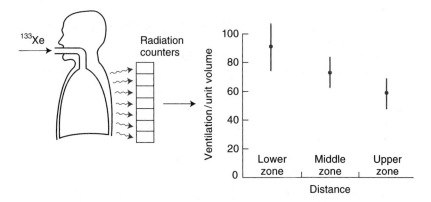

Figure 2-7. Measurement of regional differences in ventilation with radioactive xenon. When the gas is inhaled, its radiation can be detected by counters outside the chest. Note that the ventilation decreases from the lower to upper regions of the upright lung.

counting field, its radiation penetrates the chest wall and can be recorded by a bank of counters or a radiation camera. In this way, the volume of the inhaled xenon going to various regions can be determined.

Figure 2-7 shows the results obtained in a series of normal volunteers using this method. It can be seen that ventilation per unit volume is greatest near the bottom of the lung and becomes progressively smaller toward the top. Other measurements show that when the subject is in the supine position, this difference disappears with the result that apical and basal ventilations become the same. However, in that posture, the ventilation of the lowermost (posterior) lung exceeds that of the uppermost (anterior) lung. Again in the lateral position (subject on his side) the dependent lung is best ventilated. The cause of these regional differences in ventilation will be dealt with in Chapter 7.

QUESTIONS

For each question, choose the one best answer.

1. All of the following can be measured with a simple spirometer and stop-watch **EXCEPT**:
   A. Tidal volume.
   B. Functional residual capacity.
   C. Vital capacity.
   D. Total ventilation.
   E. Respiratory frequency.

2. All of the following statements about the pulmonary acinus are true **EXCEPT**:
   A. All the oxygen uptake occurs in the acini.
   B. Percentage change in volume of the acini during inspiration exceeds that of the whole lung.
   C. Volume of the acini is greater than 90% of the total volume of the lung at FRC.
   D. Each acinus is supplied by a terminal bronchiole.
   E. Acini at the base of the upright human lung at FRC are larger than those at the apex.

3. In a measurement of FRC by helium-dilution, the original and final helium concentrations were 10 and 6%, and the spirometer volume was kept at 5 liters. What was the volume of the FRC in liters?
   A. 2.5
   B. 3.0
   C. 3.3
   D. 3.8
   E. 5.0

4. A patient sits in a body plethysmograph (body box) and makes an expiratory effort against his closed glottis. What happens to the following: pressure in the lung airways, lung volume, box pressure, box volume?

	Airway Pressure	Lung Volume	Box Pressure	Box Volume
A.	↓	↑	↑	↓
B.	↓	↑	↓	↑
C.	↑	↓	↑	↓
D.	↑	↓	↓	↑
E.	↑	↑	↓	↓

5. If CO_2 production remains constant and alveolar ventilation is increased three-fold, the alveolar P_{CO_2} after a steady state is reached will be what percentage of its former value?

A. 25
B. 33
C. 50
D. 100
E. 300

6. In a measurement of physiologic dead space using Bohr's method the alveolar and mixed expired P_{CO_2} were 40 and 30 mm Hg, respectively. What was the ratio of dead space to tidal volume?

A. 0.20
B. 0.25
C. 0.30
D. 0.35
E. 0.40

3

Diffusion
How Gas Gets Across the Blood-Gas Barrier

We now consider how gases move across the blood-gas barrier by diffusion. First the basic laws of diffusion are introduced. Next we distinguish between diffusion- and perfusion-limited gases. Oxygen uptake along the pulmonary capillary is then analyzed, and there is a section on the measurement of diffusing capacity using carbon monoxide. The finite reaction rate of oxygen with hemoglobin is conveniently considered with diffusion. Finally there is a brief reference to the interpretation of measurements of diffusing capacity, and possible limitations of carbon dioxide diffusion.

In the last chapter, we looked at how gas is moved from the atmosphere to the alveoli, or in the reverse direction. We now come to the transfer of gas across the blood-gas barrier. This process occurs by *diffusion*. Only 60 years ago, some physiologists believed that the lung secreted oxygen into the capillaries, that is, the

Figure 3-1. Diffusion through a tissue sheet. The amount of gas transferred is proportional to the area (A), a diffusion constant (D), and the difference in partial pressure (P_1-P_2), and is inversely proportional to the thickness (T). The constant is proportional to the gas solubility (Sol) but inversely proportional to the square root of its molecular weight (MW).

oxygen was moved from a region of lower to one of higher partial pressure. Such a process was thought to occur in the swim bladder of fish, and it requires energy. But more accurate measurements showed that this does not occur in the lung and that all gases move across the alveolar wall by passive diffusion.

Laws of Diffusion

Diffusion through tissues is described by Fick's law (Figure 3-1). This states that the rate of transfer of a gas through a sheet of tissue is proportional to the tissue area and the difference in gas partial pressure between the two sides, and inversely proportional to the tissue thickness. As we have seen, the area of the blood-gas barrier in the lung is enormous (50 to 100 square meters), and the thickness is only $0.3\ \mu m$ in many places (Figure 1-1), so the dimensions of the barrier are ideal for diffusion. In addition, the rate of transfer is proportional to a diffusion constant which depends on the properties of the tissue and the particular gas. The constant is proportional to the solubility of the gas and inversely proportional to the square root of the molecular weight (Figure 3-1). This means that CO_2 diffuses about 20 times more rapidly than does O_2 through tissue sheets because it has a much higher solubility but not a very different molecular weight.

Fick's Law of Diffusion

- Rate of diffusion of a gas through a tissue slice is proportional to the area but inversely proportional to the thickness
- Diffusion rate is proportional to the partial pressure difference
- Diffusion rate is proportional to the solubility of the gas in the tissue but inversely proportional to the square root of the molecular weight

Diffusion and Perfusion Limitations

Suppose a red blood cell enters a pulmonary capillary of an alveolus which contains a foreign gas such as carbon monoxide or nitrous oxide. How rapidly will the partial pressure in the blood rise? Figure 3-2 shows the time courses as the red blood cell moves through the capillary, a process that takes about 3/4 sec. Look first at carbon monoxide. When the red cell enters the capillary, carbon monoxide moves rapidly across the extremely thin blood-gas barrier from the alveolar gas into the cell. As a result, the content of carbon monoxide in the cell rises. However, because of the tight bond that forms between carbon monoxide and hemoglobin within the cell, a large amount of carbon monoxide can be taken up by the cell with almost no increase in partial pressure. Thus, as the cell moves through the capillary, the carbon monoxide partial pressure in the blood hardly changes, so that no appreciable back pressure develops, and the gas continues to move rapidly across the alveolar wall. It is clear, therefore, that the amount of carbon monoxide that gets into the blood is limited by the diffusion properties of the blood-gas barrier and not by the amount of blood available.* The transfer of carbon monoxide is therefore said to be *diffusion limited*.

Contrast the time course of nitrous oxide. When this gas moves across the alveolar wall into the blood, no combination with hemoglobin takes place. As a result, the blood has nothing like the avidity for nitrous oxide that it has for carbon monoxide, and the partial pressure rises rapidly. Indeed, Figure 3-2 shows that the partial pressure of nitrous oxide in the blood has virtually reached that of the alveolar gas by the time the red cell is only one-tenth of the way along the capillary. After this point, almost no nitrous oxide is transferred. Thus, the amount of this gas taken up by the blood depends entirely on the amount of available blood flow and not at all on the diffusion properties of the blood-gas barrier. The transfer of nitrous oxide is therefore *perfusion limited*.

What of O_2? Its time course lies between those of carbon monoxide and nitrous oxide. O_2 combines with hemoglobin (unlike nitrous oxide) but with nothing like the avidity of carbon monoxide. In other words, the rise in partial pressure when O_2 enters a red blood cell is much greater than is the case for the same number of molecules of carbon monoxide. Figure 3-2 shows that the P_{O_2} of the red blood cell as it enters the capillary is already about four-tenths of the alveolar value because of the O_2 in mixed venous blood. Under typical resting conditions, the capillary P_{O_2} virtually reaches that of alveolar gas when the red cell is about one-third of the way along the capillary. Under these conditions, O_2 transfer is perfusion limited like nitrous oxide. However, in some abnormal circumstances when the diffusion properties of the lung are impaired, for example, because of thickening of the blood-gas barrier, the blood P_{O_2} does not reach the alveolar value by the end of the capillary, and now there is some diffusion limitation as well.

---

* This introductory description of carbon monoxide transfer is not completely accurate because of the rate of reaction of carbon monoxide with hemoglobin (see later).

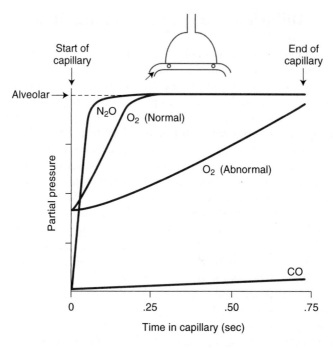

Figure 3-2. Uptake of carbon monoxide, nitrous oxide, and O_2 along the pulmonary capillary. Note that the blood partial pressure of nitrous oxide virtually reaches that of alveolar gas very early in the capillary so that the transfer of this gas is perfusion limited. By contrast, the partial pressure of carbon monoxide in the blood is almost unchanged so that its transfer is diffusion limited. O_2 transfer can be perfusion limited or partly diffusion limited, depending on the conditions.

A more detailed analysis shows that whether a gas is diffusion limited or not depends essentially on its solubility in the blood-gas barrier compared with its "solubility" in blood (actually the slope of the dissociation curve; see Chapter 6). For a gas like carbon monoxide, these are very different, whereas for a gas like nitrous oxide, they are the same. An analogy is the rate at which sheep can enter a field through a gate. If the gate is narrow but the field is large, the number of sheep that can enter in a given time is limited by the size of the gate. However, if both the gate and the field are small (or both are big) the number of sheep is limited by the size of the field.

Oxygen Uptake Along the Pulmonary Capillary

Let us take a closer look at the uptake of O_2 by blood as it moves through a pulmonary capillary. Figure 3-3A shows that the P_{O_2} in a red blood cell entering the capillary is normally about 40 mm Hg. Across the blood-gas barrier, only 0.3 μm away, is the alveolar P_{O_2} of 100 mm Hg. Oxygen floods down this large pressure gradient, and the P_{O_2} in the red cell rapidly rises; indeed, as we have seen, it very nearly reaches the P_{O_2} of alveolar gas by the time the red cell is only one-third of its way along the capillary. Thus, under normal circumstances, the difference in P_{O_2} between alveolar gas and end-capillary blood is immeasurably small—a mere fraction of a mm Hg. In other words, the diffusion reserves of the normal lung are enormous.

With severe exercise, the pulmonary blood flow is greatly increased, and the time normally spent by the red cell in the capillary, about 3/4 sec, may be reduced to as little as one-third of this. Therefore, the time available for oxygenation is less, but in normal subjects breathing air there is generally still no measurable fall in end-capillary P_{O_2}. However, if the blood-gas barrier is markedly thickened by disease so that oxygen diffusion is impeded, the rate of rise of P_{O_2} in the red blood cells is correspondingly slow, and the P_{O_2} may not reach that of alveolar gas

Figure 3-3. Oxygen time courses in the pulmonary capillary when diffusion is normal and abnormal (for example, because of thickening of the blood-gas barrier by disease). **A** shows time courses when the alveolar P_{O_2} is normal. **B** shows slower oxygenation when the alveolar P_{O_2} is abnormally low. Note that in both cases, severe exercise reduces the time available for oxygenation.

before the time available for oxygenation in the capillary has run out. In this case, a measurable difference between alveolar gas and end-capillary blood for P_{O_2} may occur.

Another way of stressing the diffusion properties of the lung is to lower the alveolar P_{O_2} (Figure 3-3B). Suppose that this has been reduced to 50 mm Hg, by the subject either going to high altitude or inhaling a low O_2 mixture. Now, although the P_{O_2} in the red cell at the start of the capillary may only be about 20 mm Hg, the partial pressure difference responsible for driving the O_2 across the blood-gas barrier has been reduced from 60 mm Hg (Figure 3-3A) to only 30 mm Hg. O_2 therefore moves across more slowly. In addition, the rate of rise of P_{O_2} for a given increase in O_2 concentration in the blood is less than it was because of the steep slope of the O_2 dissociation curve when the P_{O_2} is low (see Chapter 6). For both of these reasons, therefore, the rise in P_{O_2} along the capillary is relatively slow, and failure to reach the alveolar P_{O_2} is more likely. Thus, severe exercise at very high altitude is one of the few situations where diffusion impairment of O_2 transfer in normal subjects can be convincingly demonstrated. By the same token, patients with a thickened blood-gas barrier will be most likely to show evidence of diffusion impairment if they breathe a low oxygen mixture, especially if they exercise as well.

Diffusion of Oxygen Across the Blood-Gas Barrier

- At rest the P_{O_2} of the blood virtually reaches that of the alveolar gas after 1/3 of its time in the capillary
- Blood spends only 3/4 sec in the capillary at rest
- On exercise the time is reduced to perhaps 1/4 sec
- The diffusion process is challenged by exercise, alveolar hypoxia, and thickening of the blood-gas barrier

---

Measurement of Diffusing Capacity

We have seen that oxygen transfer into the pulmonary capillary is normally limited by the amount of blood flow available, although under some circumstances diffusion limitation also occurs (Figure 3-2). By contrast, the transfer of carbon monoxide is limited solely by diffusion, and it is therefore the gas of choice for measuring the diffusion properties of the lung. At one time O_2 was employed under hypoxic conditions (Figure 3-3B), but this technique is no longer used.

The laws of diffusion (Figure 3-1) state that the amount of gas transferred across a sheet of tissue is proportional to the area, a diffusion constant, and the difference in partial pressure, and inversely proportional to the thickness, or

$$\dot{V}gas = \frac{A}{T} \cdot D \cdot (P_1 - P_2)$$

Now for a complex structure like the blood-gas barrier of the lung, it is not possible to measure the area and thickness during life. Instead, the equation is rewritten

$$\dot{V}gas = D_L \cdot (P_1 - P_2)$$

Measurement of Diffusing Capacity

- Carbon monoxide is used because the uptake of this gas is diffusion-limited
- Normal diffusing capacity is about 25 ml.min^{-1}.mm Hg^{-1}
- Diffusing capacity increases on exercise

---

where D_L is called the *diffusing capacity of the lung* and includes the area, thickness, and diffusion properties of the sheet and the gas concerned. Thus, the diffusing capacity for carbon monoxide is given by

$$D_L = \frac{\dot{V}_{CO}}{P_1 - P_2}$$

where P_1 and P_2 are the partial pressures of alveolar gas and capillary blood, respectively. But as we have seen (Figure 3-2), the partial pressure of carbon monoxide in capillary blood is extremely small and can generally be neglected. Thus,

$$D_L = \frac{\dot{V}_{CO}}{P_{A_{CO}}}$$

or, in words, the diffusing capacity of the lung for carbon monoxide is the volume of carbon monoxide transferred in milliliters per minute per mm Hg of alveolar partial pressure.

A frequently used test is the *single breath method*, in which a single inspiration of a dilute mixture of carbon monoxide is made and the rate of disappearance of carbon monoxide from the alveolar gas during a 10-sec breathhold is calculated. This is usually done by measuring the inspired and expired concentrations of carbon monoxide with an infrared analyzer. The alveolar concentration of carbon monoxide is not constant during the breathholding period, but allowance can be made for that. Helium is also added to the inspired gas to give a measurement of lung volume by dilution.

The normal value of the diffusing capacity for carbon monoxide at rest is about 25 ml · min^{-1} · mm Hg^{-1}, and it increases to two or three times this value on exercise because of recruitment and distension of pulmonary capillaries (see Chapter 4).

Reaction Rates With Hemoglobin

So far we have assumed that all the resistance to the movement of O_2 and CO resides in the barrier between blood and gas. However, Figure 1-1 shows that the path length from the alveolar wall to the center of a red blood cell exceeds that in the wall itself, so that some of the diffusion resistance is located within the capillary. In addition, there is another type of resistance to gas transfer that is most conveniently discussed with diffusion, that is, the resistance caused by the finite rate of reaction of O_2 or CO with hemoglobin inside the red blood cell.

When O_2 (or CO) is added to blood, its combination with hemoglobin is quite fast, being well on the way to completion in 0.2 sec. However, oxygenation

occurs so rapidly in the pulmonary capillary (Figure 3-3) that even this rapid reaction significantly delays the loading of O_2 by the red cell. Thus, the uptake of
O_2 (or CO) can be regarded as occurring in two stages: (1) diffusion of O_2 through
the blood-gas barrier (including the plasma and red cell interior); and (2) reaction of the O_2 with hemoglobin (Figure 3-4). In fact, it is possible to sum the two
resultant resistances to produce an overall "diffusion" resistance.

We saw that the diffusing capacity of the lung is defined as $D_L = \dot{V}gas/(P_1 - P_2)$,
that is, as the flow of gas divided by a pressure difference. Thus, the inverse of D_L
is pressure difference divided by flow and is therefore analogous to electrical resistance. Consequently, the resistance of the blood-gas barrier in Figure 3-4 is
shown as $1/D_M$, where M means membrane. Now the rate of reaction of O_2 (or
CO) with hemoglobin can be described by θ, which gives the rate in ml per
minute of O_2 (or CO) which combine with 1 ml of blood per mm Hg partial pressure of O_2 (or CO). This is analogous to the "diffusing capacity" of 1 ml of blood
and, when multiplied by the volume of capillary blood (V_c), gives the effective
"diffusing capacity" of the rate of reaction of O_2 with hemoglobin. Again its inverse, $1/(\theta \cdot V_c)$, describes the resistance of this reaction. We can add the resistances offered by the membrane and the blood to obtain the total diffusion resistance. Thus, the complete equation is

$$\frac{1}{D_L} = \frac{1}{D_M} + \frac{1}{\theta \cdot V_c}$$

In practice, the resistances offered by the membrane and blood components are
approximately equal, so that a reduction of capillary blood volume by disease can
reduce the diffusing capacity of the lung. θ for CO is reduced if a subject breathes
a high O_2 mixture, because the O_2 competes with the CO for hemoglobin. As a
result, the measured diffusing capacity is reduced by O_2 breathing. In fact, it is
possible to separately determine D_M and V_c by measuring the diffusing capacity
for CO at different P_{O_2} values.

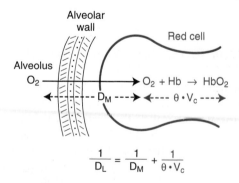

Figure 3-4. The diffusing capacity of the lung (D_L) is made up of two components,
that due to the diffusion process itself and that attributable to the time taken for
O_2 (or CO) to react with hemoglobin.

Reaction Rates of O_2 and CO with Hemoglobin

- Reaction rate of O_2 is fast but because so little time is available in the capillary, this rate can become a limiting factor
- The resistance to the uptake of O_2 attributable to reaction rate is probably about the same as that due to diffusion across the blood-gas barrier
- The reaction rate of CO can be altered by changing the alveolar P_{O_2}. In this way the separate contributions of the diffusion properties of the blood-gas barrier and the volume of capillary blood can be derived.

Interpretation of Diffusing Capacity for CO

It is clear that the measured diffusing capacity of the lung for CO depends not only on the area and thickness of the blood-gas barrier but also on the volume of blood in the pulmonary capillaries. Furthermore, in the diseased lung, the measurement is affected by the distribution of diffusion properties, alveolar volume, and capillary blood. For these reasons, the term transfer factor is sometimes used (particularly in Europe) to emphasize that the measurement does not solely reflect the diffusion properties of the lung.

CO_2 Transfer Across the Pulmonary Capillary

We have seen that diffusion of CO_2 through tissue is about 20 times faster than that of O_2 because of the much higher solubility of CO_2 (Figure 3-1). At first sight, therefore, it seems unlikely that CO_2 elimination could be affected by diffusion difficulties, and indeed this has been the general belief. However, the reaction of CO_2 with blood is complex (see Chapter 6), and although there is some uncertainty about the rates of the various reactions, it is possible that a difference between end-capillary blood and alveolar gas can develop if the blood-gas barrier is diseased.

QUESTIONS

For each question, choose the one best answer.

1. Using Fick's law of diffusion of gases through a tissue slice, if gas X is 4 times as soluble and 4 times as dense as gas Y, what is the ratio of the diffusion rates of Y to X?
   A. 0.25
   B. 0.5
   C. 2
   D. 4
   E. 8

2. An exercising subject breathes a low concentration of CO in a steady state. If the alveolar P_{CO_2} is 0.5 mm Hg and the CO uptake is 30 ml.min^{-1}, what is the diffusing capacity of the lung for CO in ml.min^{-1}.mm Hg^{-1}?
   A. 20
   B. 30

   C. 40
   D. 50
   E. 60

3. In a normal person, doubling the diffusing capacity of the lung would be expected to:
   A. Decrease arterial P_{CO_2} during resting breathing.
   B. Increase resting oxygen uptake when the subject breathes 10% oxygen.
   C. Increase the uptake of nitrous oxide during anesthesia.
   D. Increase the arterial P_{O_2} during resting breathing.
   E. Increase maximal oxygen uptake at extreme altitude.

4. A subject inhales several breaths of a gas mixture containing low concentrations of carbon monoxide and nitrous oxide. Which of the following statements is **FALSE**?
   A. The partial pressures of carbon monoxide in alveolar gas and end-capillary blood will be virtually the same.
   B. The partial pressures of nitrous oxide in alveolar gas and end-capillary blood will be virtually the same.
   C. Carbon monoxide is transferred into the blood along the whole length of the capillary.
   D. Almost all of the nitrous oxide will be taken up in the early part of the capillary.
   E. The uptake of carbon monoxide can be used to measure the diffusing capacity of the lung.

5. All of the following statements about the diffusing capacity of the lung are true **EXCEPT**:
   A. It is best measured with carbon monoxide because this gas diffuses very slowly across the blood-gas barrier.
   B. Diffusion-limitation of oxygen transfer during exercise is more likely to occur at high altitude than sea level.
   C. Breathing oxygen reduces the measured diffusing capacity for carbon monoxide compared with air breathing.
   D. It is decreased by removal of one lung.
   E. It is decreased in pulmonary fibrosis which thickens the blood-gas barrier.

6. All of the following would be expected to reduce the diffusing capacity of the lung for carbon monoxide **EXCEPT**:
   A. Emphysema which causes loss of pulmonary capillaries.
   B. Asbestosis which causes thickening of the blood-gas barrier.
   C. Pulmonary embolism which cuts off the blood supply to part of the lung.
   D. Exercise in a normal subject.
   E. Severe anemia.

Blood Flow and Metabolism
How the Pulmonary Circulation Removes Gas From the Lung and Alters Some Metabolites

4

Pressures Within Pulmonary Blood Vessels	Active Control of the Circulation
Pressures Around Pulmonary Blood Vessels	Water Balance in the Lung
Pulmonary Vascular Resistance	Other Functions of the Pulmonary Circulation
Measurement of Pulmonary Blood Flow	Metabolic Functions of the Lung
Distribution of Blood Flow	

We now turn to how the respiratory gases are removed from the lung. First the pressures inside and outside the pulmonary blood vessels are considered, and then pulmonary vascular resistance is introduced. Next we look at the measurement of total pulmonary blood flow and its uneven distribution caused by gravity. Active control of the circulation is then addressed followed by fluid balance in the lung. Finally other functions of the pulmonary circulation are dealt with, particularly the metabolic functions of the lung.

The pulmonary circulation begins at the main pulmonary artery, which receives the mixed venous blood pumped by the right ventricle. This artery then branches successively like the system of airways (Figure 1-3), and, indeed, the pulmonary arteries accompany the airways as far as the terminal bronchioles. Beyond that, they break up to supply the capillary bed which lies in the walls of the alveoli

35

(Figures 1-6 and 1-7). The pulmonary capillaries form a dense network in the alveolar wall which makes an exceedingly efficient arrangement for gas exchange (Figures 1-1, 1-6, and 1-7). So rich is the mesh that some physiologists feel that it is misleading to talk of a network of individual capillary segments and prefer to regard the capillary bed as a sheet of flowing blood interrupted in places by posts (Figure 1-6), rather like an underground parking garage. The oxygenated blood is then collected from the capillary bed by the small pulmonary veins that run between the lobules and eventually unite to form the four large veins (in humans), which drain into the left atrium.

At first sight, this circulation appears to be simply a small version of the systemic circulation which begins at the aorta and ends in the right atrium. However, there are important differences between the two circulations, and confusion frequently results from attempts to emphasize similarities between them.

Pressures Within Pulmonary Blood Vessels

The pressures in the pulmonary circulation are remarkably low. The mean pressure in the main pulmonary artery is only about 15 mm Hg; the systolic and diastolic pressures are about 25 and 8 mm Hg, respectively (Figure 4-1). The pressure is therefore very pulsatile. By contrast, the mean pressure in the aorta is about 100 mm Hg—about six times more than in the pulmonary artery. The pressures in the right and left atriums are not very dissimilar—about 2 and 5 mm Hg, respectively. Thus, the pressure differences from inlet to outlet of the pulmonary and systemic systems are about (15 − 5) = 10 and (100 − 2) = 98 mm Hg, respectively—a factor of 10.

In keeping with these low pressures, the walls of the pulmonary artery and its branches are remarkably thin and contain relatively little smooth muscle (they

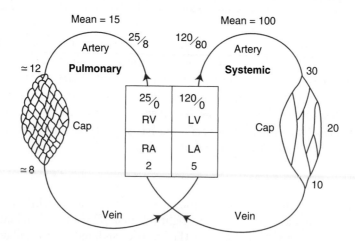

Figure 4-1. Comparison of pressures (mm Hg) in the pulmonary and systemic circulations. Hydrostatic differences modify these.

are easily mistaken for veins). This is in striking contrast to the systemic circulation where the arteries generally have thick walls and the arterioles in particular have abundant smooth muscle.

The reasons for these differences become clear when the functions of the two circulations are compared. The systemic circulation regulates the supply of blood to various organs, including those which may be far above the level of the heart (the upstretched arm, for example). By contrast, the lung is required to accept the whole of the cardiac output at all times. It is rarely concerned with directing blood from one region to another (an exception is localized alveolar hypoxia, see below), and its arterial pressure is therefore as low as is consistent with lifting blood to the top of the lung. This keeps the work of the right heart as small as is feasible for efficient gas exchange to occur in the lung.

The pressure within the pulmonary capillaries is uncertain. The best evidence suggests that it lies about halfway between pulmonary arterial and venous pressure, and probably that much of the pressure drop occurs within the capillary bed itself. Certainly the distribution of pressures along the pulmonary circulation is far more symmetrical than in its systemic counterpart, where most of the pressure drop is just upstream of the capillaries (Figure 4-1). In addition, the pressure within the pulmonary capillaries varies considerably throughout the lung because of hydrostatic effects (see below).

Pressures Around Pulmonary Blood Vessels

The pulmonary capillaries are unique in that they are virtually surrounded by gas (Figures 1-1 and 1-7). It is true that there is a very thin layer of epithelial cells lining the alveoli, but the capillaries receive little support from this and, consequently, are liable to collapse or distend, depending on the pressures within and around them. The latter is very close to alveolar pressure. (The pressure in the alveoli is usually close to atmospheric pressure; indeed, during breathholding with the glottis open, the two pressures are identical.) Under some special conditions, the effective pressure around the capillaries is reduced by the surface tension of the fluid lining the alveoli. But usually, the effective pressure is alveolar pressure, and when this rises above the pressure inside the capillaries, they collapse. The pressure difference between the inside and outside of the capillaries is often called the *transmural pressure*.

What is the pressure around the pulmonary arteries and veins? This can be considerably less than alveolar pressure. As the lung expands, these larger blood vessels are pulled open by the radial traction of the elastic lung parenchyma which surrounds them (Figures 4-2 and 4-3). Consequently, the effective pressure around them is low; in fact there is some evidence that this pressure is even less than the pressure around the whole lung (intrapleural pressure). This paradox can be explained by the mechanical advantage that develops when a relatively rigid structure like a blood vessel or bronchus is surrounded by a rapidly expanding elastic material such as lung parenchyma. In any event, both the arteries and veins increase their caliber as the lung expands.

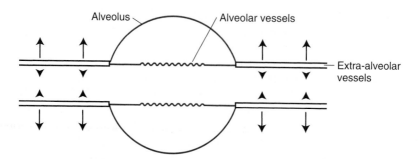

Figure 4-2. "Alveolar" and "extra-alveolar" vessels. The first are mainly the capillaries and are exposed to alveolar pressure. The second are pulled open by the radial traction of the surrounding lung parenchyma, and the effective pressure around them is therefore lower than alveolar pressure.

The behavior of the capillaries and the larger blood vessels is so different they are often referred to as alveolar and extra-alveolar vessels (Figure 4-2). Alveolar vessels are exposed to alveolar pressure and include the capillaries and the slightly larger vessels in the corners of the alveolar walls. Their caliber is determined by the relationship between alveolar pressure and the pressure within them. Extra-alveolar vessels include all the arteries and veins that run through the lung parenchyma. Their caliber is greatly affected by lung volume because this determines the expanding pull of the parenchyma on their walls. The very large vessels near the hilum are outside the lung substance and are exposed to intrapleural pressure.

Figure 4-3. Section of lung showing many alveoli and an extra-alveolar vessel (in this case, a small vein) with its perivascular sheath.

> **Alveolar and Extra-Alveolar Vessels**
> - Alveolar vessels are exposed to alveolar pressure and are compressed if this increases
> - Extra-alveolar vessels are exposed to a pressure less than alveolar, and are pulled open by the radial traction of the surrounding parenchyma

Pulmonary Vascular Resistance

It is useful to describe the resistance of a system of blood vessels as follows:

$$\text{Vascular resistance} = \frac{\text{input pressure} - \text{output pressure}}{\text{blood flow}}$$

This number is certainly not a complete description of the pressure-flow properties of the system. For example, the number usually depends on the magnitude of the blood flow. Nevertheless, it often allows a helpful comparison of different circulations or the same circulation under different conditions.

We have seen that the total pressure drop from pulmonary artery to left atrium in the pulmonary circulation is only some 10 mm Hg against about 100 mm Hg for the systemic circulation. Because the blood flows through the two circulations are virtually identical, it follows that the pulmonary vascular resistance is only one-tenth that of the systemic circulation. The pulmonary blood flow is about 6 liters/min so that, in numbers, the pulmonary vascular resistance = $(15-5)/6$ or about 1.7 mm Hg $\cdot$ liter^{-1} $\cdot$ min.* The high resistance of the systemic circulation is largely caused by very muscular arterioles which allow the regulation of blood flow to various organs of the body. The pulmonary circulation has no such vessels and appears to have as low a resistance as is compatible with distributing the blood in a thin film over a vast area in the alveolar walls.

Although the normal pulmonary vascular resistance is extraordinarily small, it has a remarkable facility for becoming even smaller as the pressure within it rises. Figure 4-4 shows that an increase in either pulmonary arterial or venous pressure causes pulmonary vascular resistance to fall. Two mechanisms are responsible for this. Under normal conditions, some capillaries are either closed, or open but with no blood flow. As the pressure rises, these vessels begin to conduct blood, thus lowering the overall resistance. This is termed *recruitment* (Figure 4-5) and is apparently the chief mechanism for the fall in pulmonary vascular resistance that occurs as the pulmonary artery pressure is raised from low levels. The reason why some vessels are unperfused at low perfusing pressures is not fully understood but perhaps is caused by random differences in the geometry of the complex network (Figure 1-3), which result in preferential channels for flow.

At higher vascular pressures, widening of individual capillary segments occurs. This increase in caliber, or *distension*, is hardly surprising in view of the very thin membrane which separates the capillary from the alveolar space (Figure 1-1). Distension is probably chiefly a change in shape of the capillaries from near-flattened

---

*Cardiologists sometimes express pulmonary vascular resistance in the units dyne $\cdot$ sec $\cdot$ cm^{-5}. The normal value is then in the region of 100.

Figure 4-4. Fall in pulmonary vascular resistance as the pulmonary arterial or venous pressure is raised. When the arterial pressure was changed, the venous pressure was held constant at 12 cm water, and when the venous pressure was changed, the arterial pressure was held at 37 cm water. (Data from an excised animal lung preparation.)

to more circular. There is evidence that the capillary wall strongly resists stretching. Distension is apparently the predominant mechanism for the fall in pulmonary vascular resistance at relatively high vascular pressures. However, recruitment and distension often occur together.

Another important determinant of pulmonary vascular resistance is *lung volume*. The caliber of the extra-alveolar vessels (Figure 4-2) is determined by a balance between various forces. As we have seen, they are pulled open as the

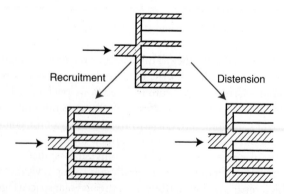

Figure 4-5. Recruitment (opening of previously closed vessels) and distension (increase in caliber of vessels). These are the two mechanisms for the decrease in pulmonary vascular resistance that occurs as vascular pressures are raised.

lung expands. As a result, their vascular resistance is low at large lung volumes. On the other hand, their walls contain smooth muscle and elastic tissue, which resist distension and tend to reduce their caliber. Consequently, they have a high resistance when lung volume is low (Figure 4-6). Indeed, if the lung is completely collapsed, the smooth muscle tone of these vessels is so effective that the pulmonary artery pressure has to be raised several centimeters of water above downstream pressure before any flow at all occurs. This is called a *critical opening pressure*.

Is the vascular resistance of the capillaries influenced by lung volume? This depends on whether alveolar pressure changes with respect to the pressure inside the capillaries, that is, whether their transmural pressure alters. If alveolar pressure rises with respect to capillary pressure, the vessels tend to be squashed, and their resistance rises. This usually occurs when a normal subject takes a deep inspiration, because the vascular pressures fall. (The heart is surrounded by intrapleural pressure, which falls on inspiration.) However, the pressures in the pulmonary circulation do not remain steady after such a maneuver. An additional factor is that the caliber of the capillaries is reduced at large lung volumes because of stretching and consequent thinning of the alveolar walls. Thus, even if the transmural pressure of the capillaries is not changed with large lung inflations, their vascular resistance increases (Figure 4-6).

Because of the role of smooth muscle in determining the caliber of the extra-alveolar vessels, drugs that cause contraction of the muscle increase pulmonary vascular resistance. These include serotonin, histamine, and norepinephrine.

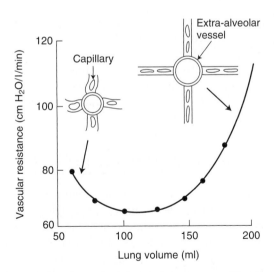

Figure 4-6. Effect of lung volume on pulmonary vascular resistance when the transmural pressure of the capillaries is held constant. At low lung volumes, resistance is high because the extra-alveolar vessels become narrow. At high volumes, the capillaries are stretched, and their caliber is reduced. (Data from an animal lobe preparation.)

Pulmonary Vascular Resistance

- Is normally very small
- Decreases on exercise because of recruitment and distention of capillaries
- Increases at high and low lung volumes
- Increases with alveolar hypoxia because of constriction of small pulmonary arteries

---

These drugs are particularly effective vasoconstrictors when the lung volume is low and the expanding forces on the vessels are weak. Drugs that can relax smooth muscle in the pulmonary circulation include acetylcholine and isoproterenol.

Measurement of Pulmonary Blood Flow

The volume of blood passing through the lungs each minute ($\dot{Q}$) can be calculated using the *Fick principle*. This states that the O_2 consumption per minute ($\dot{V}_{O_2}$) is equal to the amount of O_2 taken up by the blood in the lungs per minute. Because the O_2 concentration in the blood entering the lungs is $C\bar{v}_{O_2}$ and that in the blood leaving is Ca_{O_2} we have

$$\dot{V}_{O_2} = \dot{Q}\,(Ca_{O_2} - C\bar{v}_{O_2})$$

or

$$\dot{Q} = \frac{\dot{V}_{O_2}}{Ca_{O_2} - C\bar{v}_{O_2}}$$

$\dot{V}_{O_2}$ is measured by collecting the expired gas in a large spirometer and measuring its O_2 concentration. Mixed venous blood is taken via a catheter in the pulmonary artery, and arterial blood by puncture of the brachial or radial artery. Pulmonary blood flow can also be measured by the indicator dilution technique in which a dye or other indicator is injected into the venous circulation and its concentration in arterial blood is recorded. Both these methods are of great importance, but they will not be considered in more detail here because they fall within the province of cardiovascular physiology.

Distribution of Blood Flow

So far, we have been assuming that all parts of the pulmonary circulation behave identically. However, considerable inequality of blood flow exists within the human lung. This can be shown by a modification of the radioactive xenon method that was used to measure the distribution of ventilation (Figure 2-7). For the measurement of blood flow, the xenon is dissolved in saline and injected into a peripheral vein (Figure 4-7). When it reaches the pulmonary capillaries, it is evolved into alveolar gas because of its low solubility, and the distribution of radioactivity can be measured by counters over the chest during breathholding.

    In the upright human lung, blood flow decreases almost linearly from bottom to top, reaching very low values at the apex (Figure 4-7). This distribution is

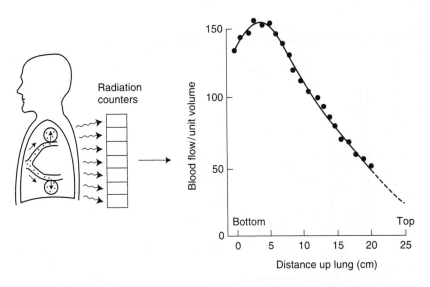

Figure 4-7. Measurement of the distribution of blood flow in the upright human lung, using radioactive xenon. The dissolved xenon is evolved into alveolar gas from the pulmonary capillaries. The units of blood flow are such that if flow were uniform, all values would be 100. Note the small flow at the apex.

affected by change of posture and exercise. When the subject lies supine, the apical zone blood flow increases but the basal zone flow remains virtually unchanged, with the result that the distribution from apex to base becomes almost uniform. However, in this posture, blood flow in the posterior (lower or dependent) regions of the lung exceeds flow in the anterior parts. Measurements on subjects suspended upside down show that apical blood flow may exceed basal flow in this position. On mild exercise, both upper and lower zone blood flows increase, and the regional differences become less.

The uneven distribution of blood flow can be explained by the hydrostatic pressure differences within the blood vessels. If we consider the pulmonary arterial system as a continuous column of blood, the difference in pressure between the top and bottom of a lung 30 cm high will be about 30 cm water, or 23 mm Hg. This is a large pressure difference for such a low-pressure system as the pulmonary circulation (Figure 4-1), and its effects on regional blood flow are shown in Figure 4-8.

There may be a region at the top of the lung (*zone 1*) where pulmonary arterial pressure falls below alveolar pressure (normally close to atmospheric pressure). If this occurs, the capillaries are squashed flat, and no flow is possible. This zone 1 does *not* occur under normal conditions because the pulmonary arterial pressure is just sufficient to raise blood to the top of the lung but may be present if the arterial pressure is reduced (following severe hemorrhage, for example) or if alveolar pressure is raised (during positive pressure ventilation). This ventilated but unperfused lung is useless for gas exchange and is called *alveolar dead space*.

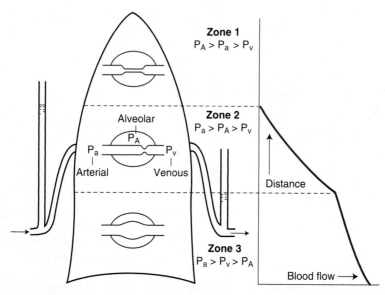

Figure 4-8. Explanation of the uneven distribution of blood flow in the lung, based on the pressures affecting the capillaries.

Farther down the lung (*zone 2*), pulmonary arterial pressure increases because of the hydrostatic effect and now exceeds alveolar pressure. However, venous pressure is still very low and is less than alveolar pressure, and this leads to remarkable pressure-flow characteristics. Under these conditions, blood flow is determined by the difference between arterial and alveolar pressures (not the usual arterial-venous pressure difference). Indeed, venous pressure has no influence on flow unless it exceeds alveolar pressure.

This behavior can be modeled with a flexible rubber tube inside a glass chamber (Figure 4-9). When chamber pressure is greater than downstream pressure, the rubber tube collapses at its downstream end, and the pressure in the tube at this point limits flow. The pulmonary capillary bed is clearly very different from a rubber tube. Nevertheless, the overall behavior is similar and is often called the Starling resistor, sluice, or waterfall effect. Because arterial pressure is increasing down the zone but alveolar pressure is the same throughout the lung, the pressure difference responsible for flow increases. In addition, increasing recruitment of capillaries occurs down this zone.

In *zone 3*, venous pressure now exceeds alveolar pressure, and flow is determined in the usual way by the arterial-venous pressure difference. The increase in blood flow down this region of the lung is apparently caused chiefly by distension of the capillaries. The pressure within them (lying between arterial and venous) increases down the zone while the pressure outside (alveolar) remains constant. Thus, their transmural pressure rises and, indeed, measurements show that their mean width increases. Recruitment of previously closed vessels may also play some part in the increase in blood flow down this zone.

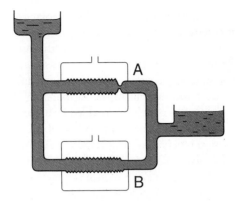

Figure 4-9. Two Starling resistors, each consisting of a thin rubber tube inside a container. When chamber pressure exceeds downstream pressure as in *A*, flow is independent of downstream pressure. However, when downstream pressure exceeds chamber pressure as in *B*, flow is determined by the upstream-downstream difference.

The scheme shown in Figure 4-8 summarizes the role played by the capillaries in determining the distribution of blood flow. At low lung volumes, the resistance of the extra-alveolar vessels becomes important, and a reduction of regional blood flow is seen, starting first at the base of the lung, where the parenchyma is least expanded (see Figure 7-8). This region of reduced blood flow is sometimes called *zone 4* and can be explained by the narrowing of the extra-alveolar vessels, which occurs when the lung around them is poorly inflated (Figure 4-6).

There are other factors causing unevenness of blood flow in the lung. In some animals, some regions of the lung appear to have an intrinsically higher vascular resistance. There is also evidence that blood flow decreases along the acinus with peripheral parts less well supplied with blood. Some measurements suggest that the peripheral regions of the whole lung receive less blood flow than the central regions. Finally, the complex, partly random arrangement of blood vessels and capillaries (Figure 1-6) causes some inequality of blood flow.

Active Control of the Circulation

We have seen that passive factors dominate the vascular resistance and the distribution of flow in the pulmonary circulation under normal conditions. However, a remarkable active response occurs when the P_{O_2} of alveolar gas is reduced. This is known as *hypoxic pulmonary vasoconstriction* and consists of contraction of smooth muscle in the walls of the small arterioles in the hypoxic region. The precise mechanism of this response is not known, but it occurs in excised isolated lung and so does not depend on central nervous connections. Excised segments of pulmonary artery can be shown to constrict if their environment is made hypoxic so that it may be a local action of the hypoxia on the artery itself. One hypothesis is that cells in the perivascular tissue release some vasoconstrictor substance in response to hypoxia, but an intensive search for the mediator has not been successful. Interestingly, it is the P_{O_2} of the alveolar gas, not the pulmonary arterial blood, that chiefly determines the response. This can be proved by perfusing a lung with blood of a high P_{O_2} while keeping the alveolar P_{O_2} low. Under these conditions the response occurs.

The vessel wall presumably becomes hypoxic through diffusion of oxygen over the very short distance from the wall to the surrounding alveoli. Recall that a small pulmonary artery is very closely surrounded by alveoli (compare the proximity of alveoli to the small pulmonary vein in Figure 4-3). The stimulus-response curve of this constriction is very nonlinear (Figure 4-10). When the alveolar P_{O_2} is altered in the region above 100 mm Hg, little change in vascular resistance is seen. However, when the alveolar P_{O_2} is reduced below approximately 70 mm Hg, marked vasoconstriction may occur, and at a very low P_{O_2} the local blood flow may be almost abolished.

The mechanism of hypoxic pulmonary vasoconstriction remains obscure in spite of a great deal of research. Recent studies suggest that inhibition of voltage-gated potassium channels and membrane depolarization may be involved, leading to increased calcium ion concentrations in the cytoplasm. An increase in cytoplasmic calcium ion concentration is the major trigger for smooth muscle contraction.

Endothelium-derived vasoactive substances play a role. Nitric oxide (NO) has been shown to be an endothelium-derived relaxing factor for blood vessels. It is formed from L-arginine via catalysis by endothelial NO synthase (eNOS) and is a final common pathway for a variety of biological processes. NO activates soluble guanylate cyclase and increases the synthesis of guanosine 3',5'-cyclic monophosphate (cyclic GMP), which leads to smooth muscle relaxation.

Figure 4-10. Effect of reducing alveolar P_{O_2} on pulmonary blood flow. (Data from anesthetized cat.)

Inhibitors of NO synthase augment hypoxic pulmonary vasoconstriction in animal preparations, and inhaled NO reduces hypoxic pulmonary vasoconstriction in humans. The required inhaled concentration of NO is extremely low (about 20 ppm), and the gas is very toxic at high concentrations. Disruption of the eNOS gene has been shown to cause pulmonary hypertension in animal models.

Pulmonary vascular endothelial cells also release potent vasoconstrictors such as endothelin-1 (ET-1) and thromboxane A_2 (TXA_2). Their roles in normal physiology and disease are the subject of intense study. Blockers of endothelin receptors have been used clinically to treat patients with pulmonary hypertension.

Hypoxic vasoconstriction has the effect of directing blood flow away from hypoxic regions of lung. These regions may result from bronchial obstruction, and by diverting blood flow the deleterious effects on gas exchange are reduced. At high altitude, generalized pulmonary vasoconstriction occurs, leading to a rise in pulmonary arterial pressure. But probably the most important situation in which this mechanism operates is at birth. During fetal life, the pulmonary vascular resistance is very high, partly because of hypoxic vasoconstriction, and only some 15% of the cardiac output goes through the lungs (see Figure 9-5). When the first breath oxygenates the alveoli, the vascular resistance falls dramatically because of relaxation of vascular smooth muscle, and the pulmonary blood flow increases enormously.

Other active responses of the pulmonary circulation have been described. A low blood pH causes vasoconstriction, especially when alveolar hypoxia is present. There is also evidence that the autonomic nervous system exerts a weak control, an increase in sympathetic outflow causing stiffening of the walls of the pulmonary arteries and vasoconstriction.

Hypoxic Pulmonary Vasoconstriction

- Alveolar hypoxia constricts small pulmonary arteries
- Probably a direct effect of the low Po_2 on vascular smooth muscle
- Critical at birth in the transition from placental to air breathing
- Directs blood flow away from poorly ventilated areas of the diseased lung in the adult

---

Water Balance in the Lung

Because only 0.3 μm of tissue separates the capillary blood from the air in the lung (Figure 1-1), the problem of keeping the alveoli free of fluid is critical. Fluid exchange across the capillary endothelium is believed to obey Starling's law. The force tending to push fluid *out* of the capillary is the capillary hydrostatic pressure minus the hydrostatic pressure in the interstitial fluid, or $P_c - P_i$. The force tending to pull fluid in is the colloid osmotic pressure of the proteins of the blood minus that of the proteins of the interstitial fluid, or $\pi_c - \pi_i$. This force depends on the reflection coefficient σ, which indicates the effectiveness of the capillary wall in preventing the passage of proteins across it. Thus,

$$\text{net fluid out} = K[(P_c - P_i) - \sigma(\pi_c - \pi_i)]$$

where K is a constant called the filtration coefficient.

Unfortunately, the practical use of this equation is limited because of our ignorance of many of the values. The colloid osmotic pressure within the capillary is about 28 mm Hg. The capillary hydrostatic pressure is probably about halfway between arterial and venous pressure but is much higher at the bottom of the lung than at the top. The colloid osmotic pressure of the interstitial fluid is not known but is about 20 mm Hg in lung lymph. However, this value may be higher than that in the interstitial fluid around the capillaries. The interstitial hydrostatic pressure is unknown, but some measurements show it is substantially below atmospheric pressure. It is probable that the net pressure of the Starling equation is outward, causing a small lymph flow of perhaps 20 ml/hr in humans under normal conditions.

Where does fluid go when it leaves the capillaries? Figure 4-11 shows that fluid which leaks out into the interstitium of the alveolar wall tracks through the interstitial space to the perivascular and peribronchial space within the lung. Numerous lymphatics run in the perivascular spaces, and these help to transport the fluid to the hilar lymph nodes. In addition, the pressure in these perivascular

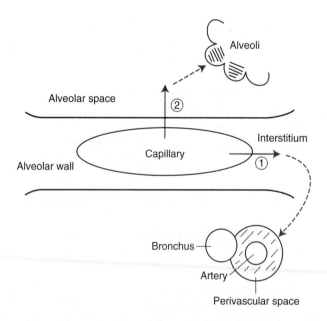

Figure 4-11. Two possible paths for fluid that moves out of pulmonary capillaries. Fluid that enters the interstitium initially finds its way into the perivascular and peribronchial spaces. Later fluid may cross the alveolar wall, filling alveolar spaces.

spaces is low, thus forming a natural sump for the drainage of fluid (compare Figure 4-2). The earliest form of pulmonary edema[†] is characterized by engorgement of these peribronchial and perivascular spaces and is known as interstitial edema. The rate of lymph flow from the lung increases considerably if the capillary pressure is raised over a long period.

In a later stage of pulmonary edema, fluid may cross the alveolar epithelium into the alveolar spaces (Figure 4-11). When this occurs, the alveoli fill with fluid one by one, and because they are then unventilated, no oxygenation of the blood passing through them is possible. What prompts fluid to start moving across into the alveolar spaces is not known, but it may be that this occurs when the maximal drainage rate through the interstitial space is exceeded and the pressure there rises too high. Fluid that reaches the alveolar spaces is actively pumped out by a sodium, potassium, ATPase pump in epithelial cells. Alveolar edema is much more serious than interstitial edema because of the interference with pulmonary gas exchange.

Other Functions of the Pulmonary Circulation

The chief function of the pulmonary circulation is to move blood to and from the blood-gas barrier so that gas exchange can occur. However, it has other important functions. One is to act as a reservoir for blood. We saw that the lung has a remarkable ability to reduce its pulmonary vascular resistance as its vascular pressures are raised through the mechanisms of recruitment and distension (Figure 4-5). The same mechanisms allow the lung to increase its blood volume with relatively small rises in pulmonary arterial or venous pressures. This occurs, for example, when a subject lies down after standing. Blood then drains from the legs into the lung.

Another function of the lung is to filter blood. Small blood thrombi are removed from the circulation before they can reach the brain or other vital organs. Many white blood cells are trapped by the lung and later released, although the value of this is not clear.

Metabolic Functions of the Lung

The lung has important metabolic functions in addition to gas exchange. A number of vasoactive substances are metabolized by the lung (Table 4-1). Because the lung is the only organ except the heart that receives the whole circulation, it is uniquely suited to modifying blood-borne substances. A substantial fraction of all the vascular endothelial cells in the body are located in the lung. The metabolic functions of the vascular endothelium are only briefly dealt with here because many fall within the province of pharmacology.

[†] For a more extensive discussion of pulmonary edema, see the companion volume, JB West: *Pulmonary Pathophysiology—The Essentials*, ed 6. Baltimore, Lippincott Williams & Wilkins, 2003.

Table 4-1. Fate of Substances in the Pulmonary Circulation

Substance	Fate
Peptides	
Angiotensin I	Converted to angiotensin II by ACE
Angiotensin II	Unaffected
Vasopressin	Unaffected
Bradykinin	Up to 80% inactivated
Amines	
Serotonin	Almost completely removed
Norepinephrine	Up to 30% removed
Histamine	Not affected
Dopamine	Not affected
Arachidonic acid metabolites	
Prostaglandin E_2 and $F_{2\alpha}$	Almost completely removed
Prostaglandin A_2	Not affected
Prostacyclin (PGI_2)	Not affected
Leukotrienes	Almost completely removed

The only known example of biological activation by passage through the pulmonary circulation is the conversion of the relatively inactive polypeptide, angiotensin I, to the potent vasoconstrictor, angiotensin II. The latter, which is up to 50 times more active than its precursor, is unaffected by passage through the lung. The conversion of angiotensin I is catalyzed by the enzyme, angiotensin-converting enzyme or ACE, which is located in small pits in the surface of the capillary endothelial cells.

Many vasoactive substances are completely or partially inactivated during passage through the lung. Bradykinin is largely inactivated (up to 80%), and the enzyme responsible is angiotensin-converting enzyme, ACE. The lung is the major site of inactivation of serotonin (5-hydroxytryptamine), but this is not by enzymatic degradation, but by an uptake and storage process (Table 4-1). Some of the serotonin may be transferred to platelets in the lung or stored in some other way and released during anaphylaxis. The prostaglandins E_1, E_2, and $F_{2\alpha}$ are also inactivated in the lung, which is a rich source of the responsible enzymes. Norepinephrine is also taken up by the lung to some extent (up to 30%). Histamine appears not to be affected by the intact lung but is readily inactivated by slices.

Some vasoactive materials pass through the lung without significant gain or loss of activity. These include epinephrine, prostaglandins A_1 and A_2, angiotensin II, and vasopressin (ADH).

Several vasoactive and bronchoactive substances are metabolized in the lung and may be released into the circulation under certain conditions. Important among these are the arachidonic acid metabolites (Figure 4-12). Arachidonic acid is formed through the action of the enzyme phospholipase A_2 on phospholipid bound to cell membranes. There are two major synthetic pathways, the initial reactions being catalyzed by the enzymes lipoxygenase and cyclooxygenase, respectively. The first produces the leukotrienes which include the mediator originally described as slow-reacting substance of anaphylaxis (SRS-A). These com-

Figure 4-12. Two pathways of arachidonic acid metabolism. The leukotrienes are generated by the lipoxygenase pathway, while the prostaglandins and thromboxane A_2 come from the cyclooxygenase pathway.

pounds cause airway constriction and may have an important role in asthma.[‡] Other leukotrienes are involved in inflammatory responses.

The prostaglandins are potent vasoconstrictors or vasodilators. PGE_2 plays an important role in the fetus because it helps to relax the patent ductus arteriosus. Prostaglandins also affect platelet aggregation and are active in other systems such as the kallikrein-kinin clotting cascade. They also may have a role in the bronchoconstriction of asthma.

There is also evidence that the lung plays a role in the clotting mechanism of blood under normal and abnormal conditions. For example, there are a large number of mast cells containing heparin in the interstitium. In addition, the lung is able to secrete special immunoglobulins, particularly IgA, in the bronchial mucus which contribute to its defenses against infection.

Synthetic functions of the lung include the synthesis of phospholipids such as dipalmitoyl phosphatidylcholine, which is a component of pulmonary surfactant (see Chapter 7). Protein synthesis is also clearly important because collagen and elastin form the structural framework of the lung. Under some conditions, proteases are apparently liberated from leukocytes in the lung, causing breakdown of collagen and elastin, and this may result in emphysema. Another significant area is carbohydrate metabolism, especially the elaboration of mucopolysaccharides of bronchial mucus.

QUESTIONS

For each question, choose the one best answer.

1. The ratio of total systemic vascular resistance to pulmonary vascular resistance is about:
   A. 2 : 1
   B. 3 : 1
   C. 5 : 1
   D. 10 : 1
   E. 20 : 1

[‡] For more details, see JB West: *Pulmonary Pathophysiology—The Essentials*, ed 6. Baltimore, Lippincott Williams & Wilkins, 2003.

2. All of the following statements about the extra-alveolar vessels of the lung are true **EXCEPT**:
   A. They are pulled open by radial traction of alveolar walls.
   B. They tend to be narrowed by smooth muscle and elastic tissue in their walls.
   C. They are exposed to alveolar pressure.
   D. On the arterial side they constrict in response to alveolar hypoxia.
   E. Their caliber is increased by lung inflation.

3. A patient with pulmonary vascular disease has mean pulmonary arterial and venous pressures of 55 and 5 mm Hg, respectively, while the cardiac output is 3 liters per minute. What is his pulmonary vascular resistance in mm Hg $\cdot$ liter$^{-1} \cdot$ min.
   A. 0.5
   B. 1.7
   C. 2.5
   D. 5
   E. 17

4. In a normal subject all of the following contribute to the fall in pulmonary vascular resistance on exercise **EXCEPT**:
   A. Increase in pulmonary arterial pressure.
   B. Increase in pulmonary venous pressure.
   C. Recruitment of pulmonary capillaries.
   D. Distension of pulmonary capillaries.
   E. Alveolar hypoxia.

5. In a measurement of cardiac output using the Fick Principle the O_2 concentrations of mixed venous and arterial blood are 16 and 20 ml $\cdot$ 100 ml^{-1}, respectively, and the O_2 consumption is 300 ml $\cdot$ min^{-1}. The cardiac output in liters $\cdot$ min^{-1} is:
   A. 2.5
   B. 5
   C. 7.5
   D. 10
   E. 75

6. In zone 2 of the lung all of the following statements are true **EXCEPT**:
   A. Arterial pressure exceeds alveolar pressure.
   B. Alveolar pressure exceeds venous pressure.
   C. Arterial pressure exceeds venous pressure.
   D. Blood flow is determined by arterial pressure minus alveolar pressure.
   E. Blood flow is determined by arterial pressure minus venous pressure.

7. Pulmonary vascular resistance is reduced by:
   A. Removal of one lung.
   B. Breathing a 10% oxygen mixture.
   C. Exhaling from functional residual capacity to residual volume.
   D. Acutely increasing pulmonary venous pressure.
   E. Mechanically ventilating the lung with positive pressure.

8. All of the following statements about hypoxic pulmonary vasoconstriction are true **EXCEPT**:
- A. It depends more on the P_{O_2} of mixed venous blood than alveolar gas.
- B. It is important in the transition from placental to air respiration.
- C. Its mechanism involves K^+ channels in vascular smooth muscle.
- D. It partly diverts blood flow from poorly ventilated regions of diseased lungs.
- E. It is reduced by inhaling low concentrations of nitric oxide.

9. If the pressure in the capillaries and interstitial space at the top of the lung are 3 and 0 mm Hg, respectively, and the colloid osmotic pressures of the blood and interstitial fluid are 25 and 5 mm Hg, respectively, what is the net pressure in mm Hg moving fluid into the capillaries?
- A. 17
- B. 20
- C. 23
- D. 27
- E. 33

10. The metabolic functions of the lung include all of the following **EXCEPT**:
- A. Converting angiotensin-1 to angiotensin-2.
- B. Inactivating bradykinin.
- C. Removing serotonin.
- D. Removing leukotrienes.
- E. Generating erythropoietin.

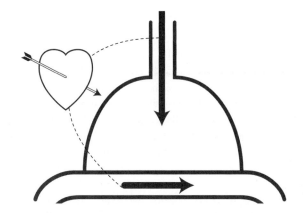

Ventilation-Perfusion Relationships

How Matching of Gas and Blood Determines Gas Exchange

5

This chapter is devoted to the primary function of the lung, that is gas exchange. First a theoretical ideal lung is considered. Then we review three mechanisms of hypoxemia including hypoventilation, diffusion limitation and shunt. The difficult concept of ventilation-perfusion inequality is then introduced, and to illustrate this the regional differences of gas exchange in the upright human lung are described. Then we examine how ventilation-perfusion inequality impairs overall gas exchange. It is emphasized that this is true not only of oxygen but also carbon dioxide. Methods of measuring ventilation-perfusion inequality are then briefly discussed.

So far we have considered the movement of air to and from the blood-gas inter-face, the diffusion of gas across it, and the movement of blood to and from the bar-rier. It would be natural to assume that if all these processes were adequate, normal gas exchange within the lung would be assured. Unfortunately, this is not so be-cause the matching of ventilation and blood flow within various regions of the lung is critical for adequate gas exchange. Indeed, mismatching of ventilation and blood flow is responsible for most of the defective gas exchange in pulmonary diseases.

In this section we shall look closely at the important (but difficult) subject of how the relations between ventilation and blood flow determine gas exchange. First, however, we shall examine two relatively simple causes of impairment of gas exchange—hypoventilation and shunt. Because all of these situations result in *hypoxemia*, that is, in an abnormally low P_{O_2} in arterial blood, it is useful to take a preliminary look at normal O_2 transfer.

Oxygen Transport From Air to Tissues

Figure 5-1 shows how the P_{O_2} falls as the gas moves from the atmosphere in which we live to the mitochondria where it is utilized. The P_{O_2} of air is 20.93% of the to-tal dry gas pressure (that is, excluding water vapor). At sea level, the barometric pressure is 760 mm Hg, and at the body temperature of 37°C, the water vapor pres-sure of moist inspired gas (which is fully saturated with water vapor) is 47 mm Hg. Thus, the P_{O_2} of inspired air is $(20.93/100) \times (760 - 47)$ or 149 mm Hg (say 150).

Figure 5-1 is drawn for a hypothetical perfect lung, and it shows that by the time the O_2 has reached the alveoli, the P_{O_2} has fallen to about 100 mm Hg, that is, by one-third. This is because the P_{O_2} of alveolar gas is determined by a balance

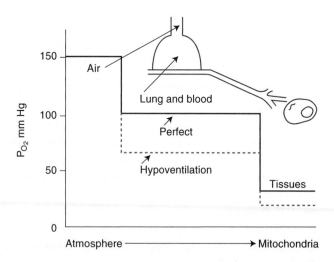

Figure 5-1. Scheme of the O_2 partial pressures from air to tissues. The *solid line* shows a hypothetical perfect situation, and the *broken line* depicts hypoventila-tion. Hypoventilation depresses the P_{O_2} in the alveolar gas and, therefore, in the tissues.

between two processes: the removal of O_2 by pulmonary capillary blood on the one hand, and its continual replenishment by alveolar ventilation on the other. (Strictly, alveolar ventilation is not continuous but is breath-by-breath. However, the fluctuation in alveolar P_{O_2} with each breath is only about 3 mm Hg, because the tidal volume is small compared with the volume of gas in the lung, so the process can be regarded as continuous.) The rate of removal of O_2 from the lung is governed by the O_2 consumption of the tissues and varies little under resting conditions. In practice, therefore, the alveolar P_{O_2} is largely determined by the level of alveolar ventilation. The same applies to the alveolar P_{CO_2}, which is normally about 40 mm Hg.

When the systemic arterial blood reaches the tissue capillaries, O_2 diffuses to the mitochondria where the P_{O_2} is much lower. The "tissue" P_{O_2} probably differs considerably throughout the body, and in some cells at least, the P_{O_2} is as low as 1 mm Hg. However, the lung is an essential link in the chain of O_2 transport, and any decrease of P_{O_2} in arterial blood must result in a lower tissue P_{O_2}, other things being equal. For the same reasons, impaired pulmonary gas exchange causes a rise in tissue P_{CO_2}.

Four Causes of Hypoxemia

- Hypoventilation
- Diffusion limitation
- Shunt
- Ventilation-perfusion inequality

Hypoventilation

We have seen that the level of alveolar P_{O_2} is determined by a balance between the rate of removal of O_2 by the blood (which is set by the metabolic demands of the tissues) and the rate of replenishment of O_2 by alveolar ventilation. Thus, if the alveolar ventilation is abnormally low, the alveolar P_{O_2} falls. For similar reasons, the P_{CO_2} rises. This is known as hypoventilation (Figure 5-1).

Causes of hypoventilation include such drugs as morphine and barbiturates which depress the central drive to the respiratory muscles, damage to the chest wall or paralysis of the respiratory muscles, and a high resistance to breathing (for example, very dense gas at great depth underwater). Hypoventilation always causes an increased alveolar and, therefore, arterial P_{CO_2}. The relationship between alveolar ventilation and P_{CO_2} was derived on p. 18:

$$P_{CO_2} = \frac{\dot{V}_{CO_2}}{\dot{V}_A} \times K$$

where $\dot{V}_{CO_2}$ is the CO_2 production, $\dot{V}_A$ is the alveolar ventilation, and K is a constant. This means that if the alveolar ventilation is halved, the P_{CO_2} is doubled, once a steady state has been established.

The relationship between the fall in P_{O_2} and the rise in P_{CO_2} that occurs in hypoventilation can be calculated from the *alveolar gas equation* if we know the composition of inspired gas and the respiratory exchange ratio R. The latter is given by the CO_2 production/O_2 consumption and is determined by the metabolism of the tissues in a steady state. It is sometimes known as the respiratory quotient. A simplified form of the alveolar gas equation is

$$P_{A_{O_2}} = P_{I_{O_2}} - \frac{P_{A_{CO_2}}}{R} + F$$

where F is a small correction factor (typically about 2 mm Hg), which we can ignore. This equation shows that if R has its normal value of 0.8, the fall in alveolar P_{O_2} is slightly greater than is the rise in P_{CO_2} during hypoventilation. The full version of the equation is given in Appendix A.

Hypoventilation always reduces the alveolar and arterial P_{O_2} except when the subject breathes an enriched O_2 mixture. In this case, the added amount of O_2 per breath can easily make up for the reduced flow of inspired gas (try question 3 on p. 72).

Hypoventilation

- Always increases the P_{CO_2}
- Decreases the P_{O_2} unless additional O_2 is inspired
- Hypoxemia is easy to reverse by adding O_2

Should alveolar ventilation be suddenly increased (for example, by voluntary hyperventilation), it may take several minutes for the alveolar P_{O_2} and P_{CO_2} to assume their new steady state values. This is because of the different O_2 and CO_2 stores in the body. The CO_2 stores are much greater than the O_2 stores because of the large amount of CO_2 in the form of bicarbonate in the blood and interstitial fluid (see Chapter 6). Therefore, the alveolar P_{CO_2} takes longer to come to equilibrium, and during the nonsteady state, the R value of expired gas is high as the CO_2 stores are washed out. Opposite changes occur with the onset of hypoventilation.

Diffusion

Figure 5-1 shows that in a perfect lung, the P_{O_2} of arterial blood would be the same as that in alveolar gas. In real life, this is not so. One reason is that although the P_{O_2} of the blood rises closer and closer to that of alveolar gas as the blood traverses the pulmonary capillary (Figure 3-3), it can never quite reach it. Under normal conditions, the P_{O_2} difference between alveolar gas and end-capillary blood resulting from incomplete diffusion is immeasurably small but is shown schematically in Figure 5-2. As we have seen, the difference can become larger during exercise, or when the blood-gas barrier is thickened, or if a low O_2 mixture is inhaled (Figure 3-3B).

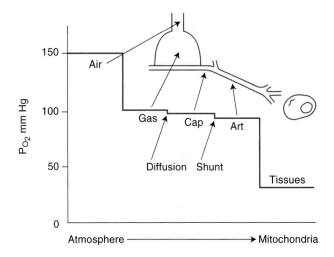

Figure 5-2. Scheme of O_2 transfer from air to tissues showing the depression of arterial P_{O_2} caused by diffusion and shunt.

Shunt

Another reason why the P_{O_2} of arterial blood is less than that in alveolar gas is shunted blood. *Shunt* refers to blood that enters the arterial system without going through ventilated areas of lung. In the normal lung, some of the bronchial artery blood is collected by the pulmonary veins after it has perfused the bronchi and its O_2 has been partly depleted. Another source is a small amount of coronary venous blood which drains directly into the cavity of the left ventricle through the Thebesian veins. The effect of the addition of this poorly oxygenated blood is to depress the arterial P_{O_2}. Some patients have an abnormal vascular connection between a small pulmonary artery and vein (pulmonary arteriovenous fistula). In patients with heart disease, there may be a direct addition of venous blood to arterial blood across a defect between the right and left sides of the heart.

When the shunt is caused by the addition of mixed venous blood to blood draining from the capillaries, it is possible to calculate the amount of the shunt flow (Figure 5-3). The total amount of O_2 leaving the system is the total blood flow $\dot{Q}_T$ multiplied by the O_2 concentration in the arterial blood Ca_{O_2}, or $\dot{Q}_T \times Ca_{O_2}$. This must equal the sum of the amounts of O_2 in the shunted blood, $\dot{Q}_S \times C\bar{v}_{O_2}$, and end-capillary blood, $(\dot{Q}_T - \dot{Q}_S) \times Cc'_{O_2}$. Thus,

$$\dot{Q}_T \times Ca_{O_2} = \dot{Q}_S \times C\bar{v}_{O_2} + (\dot{Q}_T - \dot{Q}_S) \times Cc'_{O_2}$$

Rearranging gives

$$\frac{\dot{Q}_S}{\dot{Q}_T} = \frac{Cc'_{O_2} - Ca_{O_2}}{Cc'_{O_2} - C\bar{v}_{O_2}}$$

The O_2 concentration of end-capillary blood is usually calculated from the alveolar P_{O_2} and the oxygen dissociation curve (see next chapter).

$$\frac{\dot{Q}_S}{\dot{Q}_T} = \frac{Cc'_{O_2} - Ca_{O_2}}{Cc'_{O_2} - C\bar{v}_{O_2}}$$

Figure 5-3. Measurement of shunt flow. The oxygen carried in the arterial blood equals the sum of the oxygen carried in the capillary blood and that in the shunted blood (see text).

When the shunt is caused by blood that does not have the same O_2 concentration as mixed venous blood (for example, bronchial vein blood), it is generally not possible to calculate its true magnitude. However, it is often useful to calculate an "as if" shunt, that is, what the shunt *would* be if the observed depression of arterial O_2 concentration were caused by the addition of mixed venous blood.

An important feature of a shunt is that the hypoxemia cannot be abolished by giving the subject 100% O_2 to breathe. This is because the shunted blood that bypasses ventilated alveoli is never exposed to the higher alveolar P_{O_2} so that it continues to depress the arterial P_{O_2}. However, some elevation of the arterial P_{O_2} occurs because of the O_2 added to the capillary blood of ventilated lung. Most of the added O_2 is in the dissolved form, rather than attached to hemoglobin, because the blood that is perfusing ventilated alveoli is nearly fully saturated (see next chapter). Giving the subject 100% O_2 to breathe is a very sensitive measurement of shunt because when the P_{O_2} is high, a small depression of arterial O_2 concentration causes a relatively large fall in P_{O_2} due to the almost flat slope of the O_2 dissociation curve in this region (Figure 5-4).

A shunt usually does not result in a raised P_{CO_2} in arterial blood, even though the shunted blood is rich in CO_2. The reason is that the chemoreceptors sense any elevation of arterial P_{CO_2} and they respond by increasing the ventilation. This reduces the P_{CO_2} of the unshunted blood until the arterial P_{CO_2} is normal. Indeed, in some patients with a shunt, the arterial P_{CO_2} is low because the hypoxemia increases respiratory drive (see Chapter 8).

Shunt

- Hypoxemia responds poorly to added inspired O_2
- When 100% O_2 is inspired, the arterial P_{O_2} does not rise to the expected level—a useful diagnostic test
- If the shunt is caused by mixed venous blood, its size can be calculated from the shunt equation

Figure 5-4. Depression of arterial P_{O_2} by shunt during 100% O_2 breathing. The addition of a small amount of shunted blood with its low O_2 concentration greatly reduces the P_{O_2} of arterial blood. This is because the O_2 dissociation curve is nearly flat when the P_{O_2} is very high.

The Ventilation-Perfusion Ratio

So far we have considered three of the four causes of hypoxemia: hypoventilation, diffusion, and shunt. We now come to the last cause, which is both the commonest and the most difficult to understand, namely, ventilation-perfusion inequality. It turns out that if ventilation and blood flow are mismatched in various regions of the lung, impairment of both O_2 and CO_2 transfer results. The key to understanding how this happens is the ventilation-perfusion ratio.

Consider a model of a lung unit (Figure 2-1) in which the uptake of O_2 is being mimicked using dye and water (Figure 5-5). Powdered dye is continuously poured into the unit to represent the addition of O_2 by alveolar ventilation. Water is pumped continuously through the unit to represent the blood flow which removes the O_2. A stirrer mixes the alveolar contents, a process normally accomplished by gaseous diffusion. The key question is: what determines the concentration of dye (or O_2) in the alveolar compartment and, therefore, in the effluent water (or blood)?

It is clear that both the rate at which the dye is added (ventilation) and the rate at which water is pumped (blood flow) will affect the concentration of dye in the model. What may not be intuitively clear is that the concentration of dye

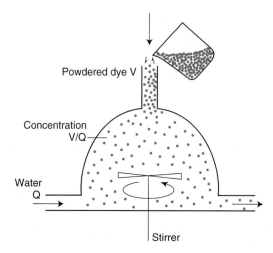

Figure 5-5. Model to illustrate how the ventilation-perfusion ratio determines the P_{O_2} in a lung unit. Powdered dye is added by ventilation at the rate V and removed by blood flow Q to represent the factors controlling alveolar P_{O_2}. The concentration of dye is given by V/Q.

is determined by the ratio of these rates. In other words, if dye is added at the rate of V gm · min^{-1} and water is pumped through at Q liters · min^{-1}, the concentration of dye in the alveolar compartment and effluent water is V/Q gm · $liter^{-1}$.

In exactly the same way, the concentration of O_2 (or better, P_{O_2}) in any lung unit is determined by the ratio of ventilation to blood flow, and not only O_2 but CO_2, N_2, and any other gas that is present under steady state conditions. This is the reason why the ventilation-perfusion ratio plays such a key role in pulmonary gas exchange.

Effect of Altering the Ventilation-Perfusion Ratio of a Lung Unit

Let us take a closer look at the way alterations in the ventilation-perfusion ratio of a lung unit affect its gas exchange. Figure 5-6A shows the P_{O_2} and P_{CO_2} in a unit with a normal ventilation-perfusion ratio (about 1—see Figure 2-1). The inspired air has a P_{O_2} of 150 mm Hg (Figure 5-1) and a P_{CO_2} of zero. The mixed venous blood entering the unit has a P_{O_2} of 40 mm Hg and P_{CO_2} of 45 mm Hg. The alveolar P_{O_2} of 100 mm Hg is determined by a balance between the addition of O_2 by ventilation and its removal by blood flow. The normal alveolar P_{CO_2} of 40 mm Hg is set similarly.

Now suppose that the ventilation-perfusion ratio of the unit is gradually reduced by obstructing its ventilation, leaving its blood flow unchanged (Figure 5-6B). It is clear that the O_2 in the unit will fall and the CO_2 will rise, although

Figure 5-6. Effect of altering the ventilation-perfusion ratio on the P_{O_2} and P_{CO_2} in a lung unit.

the relative changes of these two are not immediately obvious.* However, we can easily predict what will eventually happen when the ventilation is completely abolished (ventilation-perfusion ratio of zero). Now the O_2 and CO_2 of alveolar gas and end-capillary blood must be the same as those of mixed venous blood. (In practice, completely obstructed units eventually collapse, but we can neglect such long-term effects at the moment.) Note that we are assuming that what happens in one lung unit out of a very large number does not affect the composition of the mixed venous blood.

Suppose instead that the ventilation-perfusion ratio is increased by gradually obstructing blood flow (Figure 5-6C). Now the O_2 rises and the CO_2 falls, eventually reaching the composition of inspired gas when blood flow is abolished (ventilation-perfusion ratio of infinity). Thus, as the ventilation-perfusion ratio of the unit is altered, its gas composition approaches that of mixed venous blood or inspired gas.

A convenient way of depicting these changes is to use the O_2-CO_2 diagram (Figure 5-7). In this, P_{O_2} is plotted on the X axis, and P_{CO_2} is plotted on the Y axis. First, locate the normal alveolar gas composition, point A ($P_{O_2} = 100$, $P_{CO_2} = 40$). If we assume that blood equilibrates with alveolar gas at the end of the capillary (Figure 3-3), this point can equally well represent the end-capillary blood. Next find the

---

* The alveolar gas equation is not applicable here because the respiratory exchange ratio is not constant. The appropriate equation is

$$\frac{\dot{V}_A}{\dot{Q}} = 8.63 \cdot R \cdot \frac{(Ca_{O_2} - C\bar{v}_{O_2})}{P_{A_{CO_2}}}$$

This is called the ventilation-perfusion ratio equation.

Figure 5-7. O_2-CO_2 diagram showing a ventilation-perfusion ratio line. The P_{O_2} and P_{CO_2} of a lung unit move along this line from the mixed venous point to the inspired gas point I as its ventilation-perfusion ratio is increased (compare Figure 5-6).

mixed venous point $\bar{v}$ (P_{O_2} = 40, P_{CO_2} = 45). The bar above v means "mixed" or "mean." Finally, find the inspired point I (P_{O_2} = 150, P_{CO_2} = 0). Also, note the similarities between Figures 5-6 and 5-7.

The line joining $\bar{v}$ to I passing through A shows the changes in alveolar gas (and end-capillary blood) composition that can occur when the ventilation-perfusion ratio is either decreased below normal (A → $\bar{v}$) or increased above normal (A → I). Indeed, this line indicates *all* the possible alveolar gas compositions in a lung that is supplied with gas of composition I and blood of composition $\bar{v}$. For example, such a lung could not contain an alveolus with a P_{O_2} of 70 and P_{CO_2} of 30 mm Hg, because this point does not lie on the ventilation-perfusion line. However, this alveolar composition *could* exist if the mixed venous blood or inspired gas were changed so that the line then passed through this point.

Regional Gas Exchange in the Lung

The way in which the ventilation-perfusion ratio of a lung unit determines its gas exchange can be graphically illustrated by looking at the differences that occur down the upright lung. We saw in Figures 2-7 and 4-7 that ventilation increases slowly from top to bottom of the lung and blood flow increases more rapidly (Figure 5-8). As a consequence, the ventilation-perfusion ratio is abnormally high at the top of the lung (where the blood flow is minimal) and much lower at the bottom. We can now use these regional differences in ventilation-perfusion ratio on an O_2-CO_2 diagram (Figure 5-7) to depict the resulting differences in gas exchange.

Figure 5-9 shows the upright lung divided into imaginary horizontal "slices," each of which is located on the ventilation-perfusion line by its own ventilation-perfusion ratio. This ratio is high at the apex so that this point is found toward the right end of the line, while the base of the lung is to the left of normal (com-

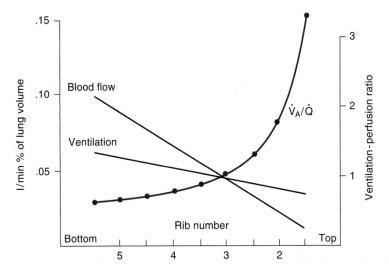

Figure 5-8. Distribution of ventilation and blood flow down the upright lung (compare Figures 2-7 and 4-7). Note that the ventilation-perfusion ratio decreases down the lung.

Figure 5-9. Result of combining the pattern of ventilation-perfusion ratio inequality shown in Figure 5-8 with the effects of this on gas exchange as shown in Figure 5-7. Note that the high ventilation-perfusion ratio at the apex results in a high P_{O_2} and low P_{CO_2} there. The opposite is seen at the base.

pare Figure 5-7). It is clear that the P_{O_2} of the alveoli (horizontal axis) decreases markedly down the lung, while the P_{CO_2} (vertical axis) increases much less.

Figure 5-10 illustrates the values that can be read off a diagram like Figure 5-9. (Of course there will be variations between individuals; the chief aim of this approach is to describe the principles underlying gas exchange.) Note first that the volume of the lung in the slices is less near the apex than the base. Ventilation is less at the top than the bottom, but the differences in blood flow are more marked. Consequently, the ventilation-perfusion ratio decreases down the lung, and all the differences in gas exchange follow from this. Note that the P_{O_2} changes by over 40 mm Hg, while the difference in P_{CO_2} between apex and base is much less. (Incidentally, the high P_{O_2} at the apex probably accounts for the preference of adult tuberculosis for this region because it provides a more favorable environment for this organism.) The variation in P_{N_2} is, in effect, by default because the total pressure in the alveolar gas is the same throughout the lung.

The regional differences in P_{O_2} and P_{CO_2} imply differences in the end-capillary concentrations of these gases, which can be obtained from the appropriate

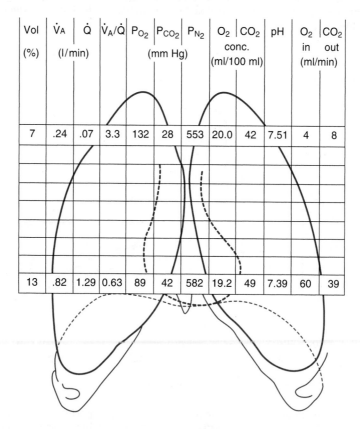

Vol (%)	V̇A (l/min)	Q̇ (l/min)	V̇A/Q̇	P_{O_2} (mm Hg)	P_{CO_2} (mm Hg)	P_{N_2} (mm Hg)	O_2 conc. (ml/100 ml)	CO_2 conc. (ml/100 ml)	pH	O_2 in (ml/min)	CO_2 out (ml/min)
7	.24	.07	3.3	132	28	553	20.0	42	7.51	4	8
13	.82	1.29	0.63	89	42	582	19.2	49	7.39	60	39

Figure 5-10. Regional differences in gas exchange down the normal lung. Only the apical and basal values are shown for clarity.

dissociation curves (Chapter 6). Note the surprisingly large difference in pH down the lung, which reflects the considerable variation in P_{CO_2} of the blood. The minimal contribution to overall O_2 uptake made by the apex can be mainly attributed to the very low blood flow there. The difference in CO_2 output between apex and base is much less because this can be shown to be more closely related to ventilation. As a result, the respiratory exchange ratio (CO_2 output/O_2 uptake) is higher at the apex than at the base. On exercise, when the distribution of blood flow becomes more uniform, the apex assumes a larger share of the O_2 uptake.

Effect of Ventilation-Perfusion Inequality on Overall Gas Exchange

While the regional differences in gas exchange discussed above are of interest, more important to the body as a whole is whether uneven ventilation and blood flow affect the overall gas exchange of the lung, that is, its ability to take up O_2 and put out CO_2. It turns out that a lung with ventilation-perfusion inequality is not able to transfer as much O_2 and CO_2 as a lung that is uniformly ventilated and perfused, other things being equal. Or if the same amounts of gas are being transferred (because these are set by the metabolic demands of the body), the lung with ventilation-perfusion inequality cannot maintain as high an arterial P_{O_2} or as low an arterial P_{CO_2} as a homogeneous lung, again other things being equal.

The reason why a lung with uneven ventilation and blood flow has difficulty oxygenating arterial blood can be illustrated by looking at the differences down the upright lung (Figure 5-11). Here the P_{O_2} at the apex is some 40 mm Hg higher than at the base of the lung. However, the major share of the blood leaving the lung comes from the lower zones, where the P_{O_2} is low. This has the result of depressing the arterial P_{O_2}. By contrast, the expired alveolar gas comes more uniformly from apex and base because the differences of ventilation are much less than those for blood flow (Figure 5-8). By the same reasoning, the arterial P_{CO_2} will be elevated because it is higher at the base of the lung than at the apex (Figure 5-10).

An additional reason why uneven ventilation and blood flow depress the arterial P_{O_2} is shown in Figure 5-12. This depicts three groups of alveoli with low, normal, and high ventilation-perfusion ratios. The O_2 concentrations of the effluent blood are 16, 19.5, and 20 ml $\cdot$ 100 ml^{-1}, respectively. As a result, the units with the high ventilation-perfusion ratio add relatively little oxygen to the blood, compared with the decrement caused by the alveoli with the low ventilation-perfusion ratio. Thus, the mixed capillary blood has a lower O_2 concentration than that from units with a normal ventilation-perfusion ratio. This can be explained by the nonlinear shape of the oxygen dissociation curve, which means that, although units with a high ventilation-perfusion ratio have a relatively high P_{O_2}, this does not increase the oxygen concentration of their blood very much. This additional reason for the depression of P_{O_2} does not apply to the elevation of the P_{CO_2} because the CO_2 dissociation curve is almost linear in the working range.

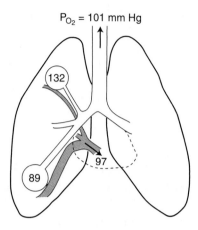

P_{O_2} = 101 mm Hg

132

97

89

Figure 5-11. Depression of the arterial P_{O_2} by ventilation-perfusion inequality. In this diagram of the upright lung, only two groups of alveoli are shown, one at the apex and another at the base. The relative sizes of the airways and blood vessels indicate their relative ventilations and blood flows. Because most of the blood comes from the poorly oxygenated base, depression of the blood P_{O_2} is inevitable.

The net result of these mechanisms is a depression of the arterial P_{O_2} below that of the mixed alveolar P_{O_2}—the so-called alveolar-arterial O_2 difference. In the normal upright lung, this difference is of trivial magnitude, being only about 4 mm Hg due to ventilation-perfusion inequality. Its development is described here only to illustrate how uneven ventilation and blood flow must result in depression of the arterial P_{O_2}. In lung disease, the lowering of arterial P_{O_2} by this mechanism can be extreme.

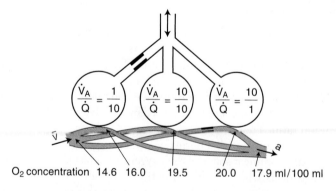

O_2 concentration 14.6 16.0   19.5   20.0   17.9 ml/100 ml

Figure 5-12. Additional reason for the depression of arterial P_{O_2} by mismatching of ventilation and blood flow. The lung units with a high ventilation-perfusion ratio add relatively little oxygen to the blood, compared with the decrement caused by alveoli with a low ventilation-perfusion ratio.

Distributions of Ventilation-Perfusion Ratios

It is possible to obtain information about the distribution of ventilation-perfusion ratios in patients with lung disease by infusing into a peripheral vein a mixture of dissolved inert gases having a range of solubilities, and measuring the concentrations of the gases in arterial blood and expired gas. The details of this technique are too complex to be described here, and it is used for research purposes rather than in the pulmonary function laboratory. The technique returns a distribution of ventilation and blood flow plotted against ventilation-perfusion ratio with 50 compartments equally spaced on a log scale.

Figure 5-13 shows a typical result from a young normal subject. Note that all the ventilation and blood flow go to compartments close to the normal ventilation-perfusion ratio of about 1.0, and, in particular, there is no blood flow to the unventilated compartment (shunt). The distributions in patients with lung disease are often very different. An example from a patient with chronic bronchitis and emphysema is shown in Figure 5-14. Note that although much of the ventilation and blood flow go to compartments with ventilation-perfusion ratios near normal, considerable blood flow is going to compartments with ventilation-perfusion ratios of between 0.03 and 0.3. Blood from these units will be poorly oxygenated and will depress the arterial P_{O_2}. There is also excessive ventilation to lung units with ventilation-perfusion ratios up to 10. These units are inefficient at eliminating CO_2. This particular patient had arterial hypoxemia but a normal arterial P_{CO_2} (see below). Other patterns are seen in other types of lung disease.

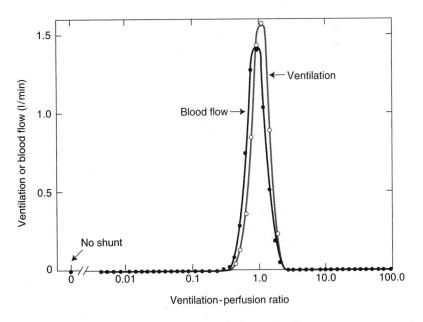

Figure 5-13. Distribution of ventilation-perfusion ratios in a young normal subject. Note the narrow dispersion and absence of shunt.

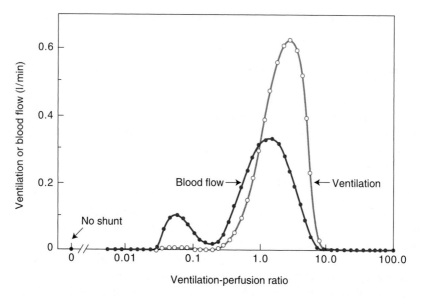

Figure 5-14. Distribution of ventilation-perfusion ratios in a patient with chronic bronchitis and emphysema. Note particularly the blood flow to lung units with very low ventilation-perfusion ratios.

Ventilation-Perfusion Inequality as a Cause of CO_2 Retention

Imagine a lung that is uniformly ventilated and perfused and that is transferring normal amounts of O_2 and CO_2. Suppose that in some magical way, the matching of ventilation and blood flow is suddenly disturbed while everything else remains unchanged. What happens to gas exchange? It transpires that the effect of this "pure" ventilation-perfusion inequality (that is, everything else held constant) is to reduce *both* the O_2 uptake and CO_2 output of the lung. In other words, the lung becomes less efficient as a gas exchanger for both gases. Hence, mismatching ventilation and blood flow must cause both hypoxemia and hypercapnia (CO_2 retention), other things being equal.

However, in practice, patients with undoubted ventilation-perfusion inequality often have a normal arterial P_{CO_2}. The reason for this is that whenever the chemoreceptors sense a rising P_{CO_2}, there is an increase in ventilatory drive (Chapter 8). The consequent increase in ventilation to the alveoli is usually effective in returning the arterial P_{CO_2} to normal. However, such patients can only maintain a normal P_{CO_2} at the expense of this increased ventilation to their alveoli; the ventilation in excess of what they would normally require is sometimes referred to as *wasted ventilation* and is necessary because the lung units with abnormally high ventilation-perfusion ratios are inefficient at eliminating CO_2. Such units are said to constitute an *alveolar dead space*.

Ventilation-Perfusion Inequality

- The ventilation-perfusion ratio ($\dot{V}A/\dot{Q}$) determines the gas exchange in any single lung unit
- Regional differences of $\dot{V}A/\dot{Q}$ in the upright human lung cause a pattern of regional gas exchange
- $\dot{V}A/\dot{Q}$ inequality impairs the uptake or elimination of all gases by the lung
- Although the elimination of CO_2 is impaired by $\dot{V}A/\dot{Q}$ inequality, this can be corrected by increasing the ventilation to the alveoli
- By contrast, the hypoxemia resulting from $\dot{V}A/\dot{Q}$ inequality cannot be eliminated by increases in ventilation
- The different behavior of the two gases results from the different shapes of their dissociation curves

---

While the increase in ventilation to a lung with ventilation-perfusion inequality is usually effective at reducing the arterial P_{CO_2}, it is much less effective at increasing the arterial P_{O_2}. The reason for the different behavior of the two gases lies in the shapes of the CO_2 and O_2 dissociation curves (Chapter 6). The CO_2 dissociation curve is almost straight in the physiological range, with the result that an increase in ventilation will raise the CO_2 output of lung units with both high and low ventilation-perfusion ratios. By contrast, the almost flat top of the O_2 dissociation curve means that only units with moderately low ventilation-perfusion ratios will benefit appreciably from the increased ventilation. Those units that are very high on the dissociation curve (high ventilation-perfusion ratio) increase the O_2 concentration of their effluent blood very little (Figure 5-12). Those units which have a very low ventilation-perfusion ratio continue to put out blood with an O_2 concentration close to that of mixed venous blood. The net result is that the mixed arterial P_{O_2} rises only modestly, and some hypoxemia always remains.

Measurement of Ventilation-Perfusion Inequality

How can we assess the amount of ventilation-perfusion inequality in diseased lungs? Radioactive gases can be used to define topographical differences in ventilation and blood flow in the normal upright lung (Figures 2-7 and 4-7), but in most patients large amounts of inequality exist between closely adjacent units, and this cannot be distinguished by counters over the chest. In practice, we turn to indices based on the resulting impairment of gas exchange.[†]

One useful measurement is the *alveolar-arterial* P_{O_2} *difference*, obtained by subtracting the arterial P_{O_2} from the so-called "ideal" alveolar P_{O_2}. The latter is the P_{O_2} which the lung *would* have if there were no ventilation-perfusion inequality

---

[†] For more details of this difficult subject, see JB West: *Pulmonary Pathophysiology— The Essentials*, ed 6. Baltimore, Lippincott Williams & Wilkins, 2003.

and it was exchanging gas at the same respiratory exchange ratio as the real lung. It is derived from the alveolar gas equation:

$$P_{AO_2} = P_{IO_2} - \frac{P_{ACO_2}}{R} + F$$

The arterial P_{CO_2} is used for the alveolar value.

An example will clarify this. Suppose a patient who is breathing air at sea level has an arterial P_{O_2} of 50 mm Hg, an arterial P_{CO_2} of 60 mm Hg, and R is 0.8. Could the arterial hypoxemia be explained by hypoventilation?

From the alveolar gas equation, the ideal alveolar P_{O_2} is given by

$$P_{AO_2} = 149 - \frac{60}{0.8} + F = 74 \text{ mm Hg}$$

where the inspired P_{O_2} is 149 mm Hg and we ignore the small factor F. Thus, the alveolar-arterial P_{O_2} difference is approximately $(74 - 50) = 24$ mm Hg. This is abnormally high, and indicates that there is ventilation-perfusion inequality.

Additional information on the measurement of ventilation-perfusion inequality can be found in Chapter 10.

QUESTIONS

For each question, choose the one best answer.

1. A climber reaches an altitude of 4500 m (14,800 ft) where the barometric pressure is 447 mm Hg. The P_{O_2} of moist inspired gas (in mm Hg) is:
    A. 47
    B. 63
    C. 75
    D. 84
    E. 98

2. A man with normal lungs and an arterial P_{CO_2} of 40 mm Hg takes an overdose of barbiturate which halves his alveolar ventilation but does not change his CO_2 output. If his respiratory exchange ratio is 0.8, what will be his arterial P_{O_2} (in mm Hg) approximately?
    A. 40
    B. 50
    C. 60
    D. 70
    E. 80

3. In the situation described in Question 2 how much does the inspired O_2 concentration (%) have to be raised to return the arterial P_{O_2} to its original level?
    A. 7
    B. 11
    C. 15
    D. 19
    E. 23

4. A patient with normal lungs but a right-to-left shunt is found at catheterization to have oxygen concentrations in his arterial and mixed venous blood of

18 and 14 ml · 100 ml^{-1}, respectively. If the O_2 concentration of the blood leaving the pulmonary capillaries is calculated to be 20 ml · 100 ml^{-1}, what is his shunt as a percentage of his cardiac output?

A. 23
B. 33
C. 43
D. 53
E. 63

5. If a climber on the summit of Mt. Everest (barometric pressure 247 mm Hg) maintains an alveolar Po_2 of 34 mm Hg and is in a steady state (R ≤ 1), his alveolar Pco_2 (in mm Hg) cannot be any higher than:

A. 5
B. 8
C. 10
D. 12
E. 15

6. A patient with severe chronic obstructive pulmonary disease, which causes marked ventilation-perfusion inequality, has an arterial Po_2 of 50 mm Hg and an arterial Pco_2 of 40 mm Hg. The Pco_2 is normal despite the hypoxemia because:

A. Ventilation-perfusion inequality does not interfere with CO_2 elimination.
B. Much of the CO_2 is carried as bicarbonate.
C. The formation of carbonic acid is accelerated by carbonic anhydrase.
D. CO_2 diffuses much faster through tissue than O_2.
E. The O_2 and CO_2 dissociation curves have different shapes.

7. The apex of the upright human lung compared with the base has a:

A. Higher Po_2.
B. Higher ventilation.
C. Lower pH in end-capillary blood.
D. Higher blood flow.
E. Smaller alveoli.

8. If the ventilation-perfusion ratio of a lung unit is decreased by partial bronchial obstruction while the rest of the lung is unaltered, the affected lung unit will show:

A. Increased alveolar Po_2.
B. Decreased alveolar Pco_2.
C. No change in alveolar PN_2.
D. Rise in pH of end-capillary blood.
E. Fall in oxygen uptake.

9. A patient with lung disease who is breathing air has an arterial Po_2 and Pco_2 of 49 and 48 mm Hg, respectively, and a respiratory exchange ratio of 0.8. The approximate alveolar-arterial difference for Po_2 (in mm Hg) is:

A. 10
B. 20
C. 30
D. 40
E. 50

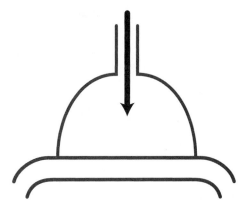

6

Gas Transport by the Blood
How Gases Are Moved to the Peripheral Tissues

Oxygen	**Acid-Base Status**
Dissolved O_2	Respiratory Acidosis
Hemoglobin	Respiratory Alkalosis
O_2 Dissociation Curve	Metabolic Acidosis
Carbon Dioxide	Metabolic Alkalosis
CO_2 Carriage	**Blood-Tissue Gas Exchange**
CO_2 Dissociation Curve	

We now consider the carriage of the respiratory gases, oxygen and carbon dioxide, by the blood. First we look at the oxygen dissociation curve including the factors that affect the oxygen affinity of hemoglobin. Then we turn to carbon dioxide which is carried in the blood in three forms. Next we consider the acid-base status of the blood and the four principal abnormalities: respiratory acidosis and alkalosis, and metabolic acidosis and alkalosis. Finally we briefly look at gas exchange in peripheral tissues.

Oxygen

O_2 is carried in the blood in two forms: dissolved and combined with hemoglobin.

Figure 6-1. O_2 dissociation curve (*solid line*) for pH 7.4, P_{CO_2} 40 mm Hg, and 37°C. The total blood O_2 concentration is also shown for a hemoglobin concentration of 15 gm · 100 ml^{-1} of blood.

Dissolved O$_2$

This obeys Henry's law, that is, the amount dissolved is proportional to the partial pressure (Figure 6-1). For each mm Hg of P_{O_2} there is 0.003 ml O_2 · 100 ml^{-1} of blood (sometimes written 0.003 vol %). Thus, normal arterial blood with a P_{O_2} of 100 mm Hg contains 0.3 ml O_2 · 100 ml^{-1}.

It is easy to see that this way of transporting O_2 must be inadequate. Suppose that the cardiac output during strenuous exercise is 30 liters · min^{-1}. Because arterial blood contains 0.3 ml O_2 · 100 ml^{-1} blood (that is, 3 ml O_2 · liter^{-1} blood) as dissolved O_2, the total amount delivered to the tissues is only 30 × 3 = 90 ml · min^{-1}. However, the tissue requirements may be as high as 3000 ml O_2 · min^{-1}. Clearly, an additional method of transporting O_2 is required.

Hemoglobin

Heme is an iron-porphyrin compound, and this is joined to the protein globin which consists of four polypeptide chains. The chains are of two types, alpha and beta, and differences in their amino acid sequences give rise to various types of human hemoglobin. Normal adult hemoglobin is known as A. Hemoglobin F (fetal) makes up part of the hemoglobin of the newborn infant and is gradually replaced over the first year or so of postnatal life. Hemoglobin S (sickle) has valine instead of glutamic acid in the beta chains. This results in a shift in the dissociation curve to the right, but, more important, the deoxygenated form is poorly soluble and crystallizes within the red cell. As a consequence, the cell shape changes from biconcave to crescent or sickle shaped with increased fragility and a tendency to thrombus formation. Many other varieties of hemoglobin have now been described, some with bizarre O_2 affinities. For more information about hemoglobin, consult a textbook of biochemistry.

Normal hemoglobin A can have its ferrous ion oxidized to the ferric form by various drugs and chemicals, including nitrites, sulfonamides, and acetanilid. This ferric form is known as methemoglobin. There is a congenital cause in which the enzyme methemoglobin reductase is deficient within the red blood cell. Another abnormal form is sulfhemoglobin. These compounds are not useful for O_2 carriage.

O_2 Dissociation Curve

O_2 forms an easily reversible combination with hemoglobin (Hb) to give oxyhemoglobin: $O_2 + Hb \rightleftharpoons HbO_2$. Suppose we take a number of glass containers (tonometers), each containing a small volume of blood, and add gas with various concentrations of O_2. After allowing time for the gas and blood to reach equilibrium, we measure the P_{O_2} of the gas and the O_2 concentration of the blood. Knowing that 0.003 ml O_2 will be dissolved in each 100 ml of blood/mm Hg P_{O_2}, we can calculate the O_2 combined with Hb (Figure 6-1). Note that the amount of O_2 carried by the Hb increases rapidly up to a P_{O_2} of about 50 mm Hg, but above that the curve becomes much flatter.

The maximum amount of O_2 that can be combined with Hb is called the O_2 *capacity*. This is when all the available binding sites are occupied by O_2. It can be measured by exposing the blood to a very high P_{O_2} (say 600 mm Hg) and subtracting the dissolved O_2. One gram of pure Hb can combine with 1.39* ml O_2, and because normal blood has about 15 gm of Hb $\cdot$ 100 ml^{-1}, the O_2 capacity is about 20.8 ml $O_2 \cdot$ 100 ml^{-1} of blood.

The O_2 *saturation* of Hb is the percentage of the available binding sites that have O_2 attached, and is given by

$$\frac{O_2 \text{ combined with Hb}}{O_2 \text{ capacity}} \times 100$$

The O_2 saturation of arterial blood with P_{O_2} of 100 mm Hg is about 97.5%, while that of mixed venous blood with a P_{O_2} of 40 mm Hg is about 75%.

The change in Hb from the fully oxygenated state to its deoxygenated state is accompanied by a conformational change in the molecule. The oxygenated form is the R (relaxed) state, while the deoxy form is the T (tense) state. It is important to grasp the relationships between P_{O_2}, O_2 saturation, and O_2 concentration (Figure 6-2). For example, suppose a severely anemic patient with an Hb concentration of only 10 gm $\cdot$ 100 ml^{-1} of blood has normal lungs and an arterial P_{O_2} of 100 mm Hg. This patient's O_2 capacity will be $20.8 \times 10/15 = 13.9$ ml $\cdot$ 100 ml^{-1}. The patient's O_2 saturation will be 97.5% (at normal pH, P_{CO_2}, and temperature), but

---

*Some measurements give 1.34 or 1.36 ml. The reason is that under the normal conditions of the body, some of the hemoglobin is in forms such as methemoglobin that cannot combine with O_2.

Figure 6-2. Effects of anemia and polycythemia on O_2 concentration and saturation. In addition, the *broken line* shows the O_2 dissociation curve when one-third of the normal hemoglobin is bound to CO. Note that the curve is shifted to the left.

the O_2 combined with Hb will be only 13.5 ml · 100 ml^{-1}. Dissolved O_2 will contribute 0.3 ml, giving a total O_2 concentration of 13.8 ml · 100 ml^{-1} of blood. In general, the oxygen concentration of blood (in ml O_2 · 100 ml^{-1} blood) is given by

$$\left(1.39 \times Hb \times \frac{Sat}{100}\right) + 0.003 \, P_{O_2}$$

where Hb is the hemoglobin concentration in gm · 100 ml^{-1}, Sat is the percentage saturation of the hemoglobin, and P_{O_2} is in mm Hg.

The curved shape of the O_2 dissociation curve has several physiological advantages. The flat upper portion means that even if the P_{O_2} in alveolar gas falls somewhat, loading of O_2 will be little affected. In addition, as the red cell takes up O_2 along the pulmonary capillary (Figure 3-3), a large partial pressure difference between alveolar gas and blood continues to exist when most of the O_2 has been transferred. As a result, the diffusion process is hastened. The steep lower part of the dissociation curve means that the peripheral tissues can withdraw large amounts of O_2 for only a small drop in capillary P_{O_2}. This maintenance of blood P_{O_2} assists the diffusion of O_2 into the tissue cells.

Because reduced Hb is purple, a low arterial O_2 saturation causes *cyanosis*. However, this is not a reliable sign of mild desaturation because its recognition depends on so many variables, such as lighting conditions and skin pigmentation. Because it is the amount of reduced Hb that is important, cyanosis is often marked when polycythemia is present but is difficult to detect in anemic patients.

The O_2 dissociation curve is shifted to the right, i.e., the O_2 affinity of Hb is reduced, by an increase in H$^+$ concentration, P_{CO_2}, temperature, and the con-

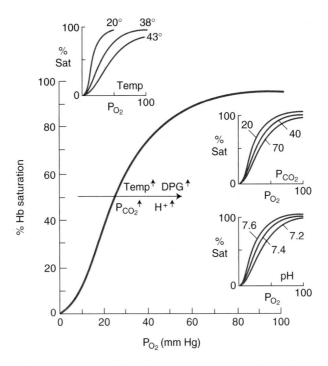

Figure 6-3. Rightward shift of the O_2 dissociation curve by increase of H^+, P_{CO_2}, temperature, and 2,3-diphosphoglycerate (DPG).

centration of 2,3-diphosphoglycerate in the red cells (Figure 6-3). Opposite changes shift it to the left. Most of the effect of P_{CO_2}, which is known as the *Bohr effect*, can be attributed to its action on H^+ concentration. A rightward shift means more unloading of O_2 at a given P_{O_2} in a tissue capillary. A simple way to remember these shifts is that an exercising muscle is acid, hypercarbic, and hot, and it benefits from increased unloading of O_2 from its capillaries.

The environment of the Hb within the red cell also affects the O_2 dissociation curve. An increase in 2,3-diphosphoglycerate (DPG), which is an end-product of red cell metabolism, shifts the curve to the right. An increase in concentration of this material occurs in chronic hypoxia, for example, at high altitude or in the presence of chronic lung disease. As a result, the unloading of O_2 to peripheral tissues is assisted. By contrast, stored blood in a blood bank may be depleted of

---

Oxygen Dissociation Curve

- Useful "anchor" points: P_{O_2} 40, S_{O_2} 75%; P_{O_2} 100, S_{O_2} 97%
- Curve is right-shifted by increases in temperature, P_{CO_2}, H^+, 2,3 DPG
- Small addition of CO to blood causes a left shift

2,3-DPG, and unloading of O_2 is therefore impaired. A useful measure of the position of the dissociation curve is the P_{O_2} for 50% O_2 saturation. This is known as the P_{50}. The normal value for human blood is about 27 mm Hg.

Carbon monoxide interferes with the O_2 transport function of blood by combining with Hb to form carboxyhemoglobin (COHb). CO has about 240 times the affinity of O_2 for Hb; this means that CO will combine with the same amount of Hb as O_2 when the CO partial pressure is 240 times lower. In fact, the CO dissociation curve is almost identical in shape to the O_2 dissociation curve of Figure 6-3, except that the P_{CO} axis is greatly compressed. For example, at a P_{CO} of 0.16 mm Hg, 75% of the Hb is combined with CO as COHb. For this reason, small amounts of CO can tie up a large proportion of the Hb in the blood, thus making it unavailable for O_2 carriage. If this happens, the Hb concentration and P_{O_2} of blood may be normal, but its O_2 concentration is grossly reduced. The presence of COHb also shifts the O_2 dissociation curve to the left (Figure 6-2), thus interfering with the unloading of O_2. This is an additional feature of the toxicity of CO.

Carbon Dioxide

CO_2 Carriage

CO_2 is carried in the blood in three forms: dissolved, as bicarbonate, and in combination with proteins as carbamino compounds (Figure 6-4).

Dissolved CO_2, like O_2, obeys Henry's law, but CO_2 is about 20 times more soluble than O_2. As a result, dissolved CO_2 plays a significant role in its carriage in

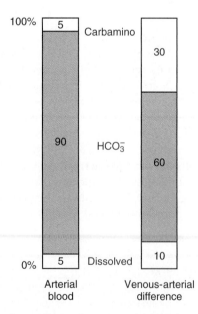

Figure 6-4. The *first column* shows the proportions of the total CO_2 concentration in arterial blood. The *second column* shows the proportions that make up the venous-arterial difference.

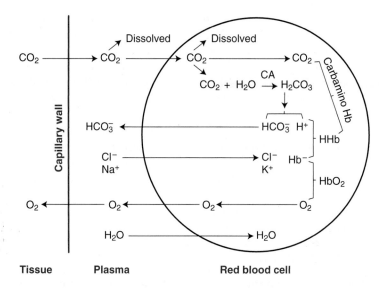

Figure 6-5. Scheme of the uptake of CO_2 and liberation of O_2 in systemic capillaries. Exactly opposite events occur in the pulmonary capillaries.

that about 10% of the gas that is evolved into the lung from the blood is in the dissolved form (Figure 6-4).

Bicarbonate is formed in blood by the following sequence:

$$CO_2 + H_2O \overset{CA}{\rightleftharpoons} H_2CO_3 \rightleftharpoons H^+ + HCO_3^-$$

The first reaction is very slow in plasma but fast within the red blood cell because of the presence there of the enzyme *carbonic anhydrase* (CA). The second reaction, ionic dissociation of carbonic acid, is fast without an enzyme. When the concentration of these ions rises within the red cell, HCO_3^- diffuses out but H^+ cannot easily do this because the cell membrane is relatively impermeable to cations. Thus, to maintain electrical neutrality, Cl^- ions move into the cell from the plasma, the so-called *chloride shift* (Figure 6-5). The movement of chloride is in accordance with the Gibbs-Donnan equilibrium.

Some of the H^+ ions liberated are bound to reduced hemoglobin:

$$H^+ + HbO_2 \rightleftharpoons H^+ \cdot Hb + O_2$$

This occurs because reduced Hb is less acid (that is, a better proton acceptor) than the oxygenated form. Thus, the presence of reduced Hb in the peripheral blood helps with the loading of CO_2, while the oxygenation that occurs in the pulmonary capillary assists in the unloading. The fact that deoxygenation of the blood increases its ability to carry CO_2 is known as the *Haldane effect*.

These events associated with the uptake of CO_2 by blood increase the osmolar content of the red cell, and, consequently, water enters the cell, thus increasing its volume. When the cells pass through the lung, they shrink a little.

Carbamino compounds are formed by the combination of CO_2 with terminal amine groups in blood proteins. The most important protein is the globin of hemoglobin: $Hb·NH_2 + CO_2 \rightleftharpoons Hb·NH·COOH$, giving carbamino-hemoglobin. This reaction occurs rapidly without an enzyme, and reduced Hb can bind more CO_2 as carbamino-hemoglobin than HbO_2. Thus, again unloading of O_2 in peripheral capillaries facilitates the loading of CO_2, while oxygenation has the opposite effect.

The relative contributions of the various forms of CO_2 in blood to the total CO_2 concentration are summarized in Figure 6-4. Note that the great bulk of the CO_2 is in the form of bicarbonate. The amount dissolved is small, as is that in the form of carbamino-hemoglobin. However, these proportions do not reflect the changes that take place when CO_2 is loaded or unloaded by the blood. Of the total venous-arterial difference, about 60% is attributable to HCO_3^-, 30% to carbamino compounds, and 10% to dissolved CO_2.

CO_2 Dissociation Curve

The relationship between the P_{CO_2} and the total CO_2 concentration of blood is shown in Figure 6-6. Note that the CO_2 dissociation curve is much more linear than is the O_2 dissociation curve (Figure 6-1). Note also that the lower the saturation of Hb with O_2, the larger the CO_2 concentration for a given P_{CO_2}. As we have seen, this *Haldane effect* can be explained by the better ability of reduced Hb to mop up the H^+ ions produced when carbonic acid dissociates, and the greater facility of reduced Hb to form carbamino-hemoglobin. Figure 6-7 shows that the CO_2 dissociation curve is considerably steeper than that for O_2. For example, in the range of 40 to 50 mm Hg, the CO_2 concentra-

Figure 6-6. CO_2 dissociation curves for blood of different O_2 saturations. Note that oxygenated blood carries less CO_2 for the same P_{CO_2}. The *inset* shows the "physiological" curve between arterial and mixed venous blood.

Figure 6-7. Typical O_2 and CO_2 dissociation curves plotted with the same scales. Note that the CO_2 curve is much steeper.

tion changes by about 4.7, compared with an O_2 concentration of only about 1.7 ml/100 ml. This is why the Po_2 difference between arterial and mixed venous blood is large (typically about 60 mm Hg) but the Pco_2 difference is small (about 5 mm Hg).

Carbon Dioxide Dissociation Curve

- CO_2 carried as: dissolved, bicarbonate, carbamino
- CO_2 curve is steeper and more linear than the O_2 curve
- CO_2 curve is right-shifted by increases in So_2

Acid-Base Status

The transport of CO_2 has a profound effect on the acid-base status of the blood and the body as a whole. The lung excretes over 10,000 mEq of carbonic acid per day compared with less than 100 mEq of fixed acids by the kidney. Therefore, by altering alveolar ventilation and thus the elimination of CO_2, the body has great control over its acid-base balance. This subject will be treated only briefly here because it overlaps the area of renal physiology.

The pH resulting from the solution of CO_2 in blood and the consequent dissociation of carbonic acid is given by the Henderson-Hasselbalch equation. It is derived as follows. In the equation

$$H_2CO_3 \rightleftharpoons H^+ + HCO_3^-$$

the law of the mass action gives the dissociation constant of carbonic acid K'_A as

$$\frac{(H^+) \times (HCO_3^-)}{(H_2CO_3)}$$

Because the concentration of carbonic acid is proportional to the concentration of dissolved carbon dioxide, we can change the constant and write

$$K_A = \frac{(H^+) \times (HCO_3^-)}{(CO_2)}$$

Taking logarithms

$$\log K_A = \log (H^+) + \log \frac{(HCO_3^-)}{(CO_2)}$$

whence

$$-\log (H^+) = -\log K_A + \log \frac{(HCO_3^-)}{(CO_2)}$$

Because pH is the negative logarithm

$$pH = pK_A + \log \frac{(HCO_3^-)}{(CO_2)}$$

Because CO_2 obeys Henry's law, the CO_2 concentration (in mmol/liter) can be replaced by $(P_{CO_2} \times 0.03)$. The equation then becomes

$$pH = pK_A + \log \frac{(HCO_3^-)}{0.03\ P_{CO_2}}$$

The value of pK_A is 6.1, and the normal HCO_3^- concentration in arterial blood is 24 mmol/liter. Substituting gives

$$pH = 6.1 + \log \frac{24}{0.03 \times 40}$$

$$= 6.1 + \log 20$$
$$= 6.1 + 1.3$$

Therefore, $pH = 7.4$

Note that as long as the ratio of bicarbonate concentration to $(P_{CO_2} \times 0.03)$ remains equal to 20, the pH will remain at 7.4. The bicarbonate concentration is determined chiefly by the kidney and the P_{CO_2} by the lung.

The relationships between pH, P_{CO_2}, and HCO_3^- are conveniently shown on a Davenport diagram (Figure 6-8). The two axes show HCO_3^- and pH, and lines of equal P_{CO_2} sweep across the diagram. Normal plasma is represented by point A. The line CAB shows the relationship between HCO_3^- and pH as carbonic acid is added to whole blood, that is, it is part of the titration curve for blood and is called the *buffer line*. The slope of this line is steeper than that measured in plasma separated from blood because of the presence of hemoglobin, which has an additional buffering action. The slope of the line measured on whole blood *in vitro* is usually a little different from that found in a patient because of the buffering action of the interstitial fluid and other body tissues.

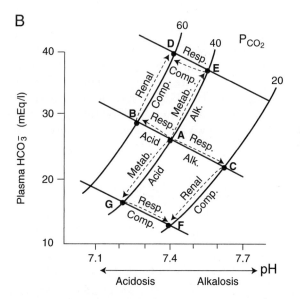

Figure 6-8. Davenport diagram showing the relationships among HCO⁻₃, pH, and P$_{CO_2}$. **A** shows the normal buffer line BAC. **B** shows the changes occurring in respiratory and metabolic acidosis and alkalosis (see text). The vertical distance between buffer lines is the *base excess.*

If the plasma bicarbonate concentration is altered by the kidney, the buffer line is displaced. An increase in bicarbonate concentration displaces the buffer line upward as shown, for example, by line DE in Figure 6-8. In this case, the *base excess* is increased and is given by the vertical distance between the two buffer lines DE and BAC. By contrast, a reduced bicarbonate concentration displaces the buffer line downward (line GF), and there is now a negative base excess, or *base deficit*.

The ratio of bicarbonate to P_{CO_2} can be disturbed in four ways: both P_{CO_2} and bicarbonate can be raised or lowered. Each of these four disturbances gives rise to a characteristic acid-base change.

Respiratory Acidosis

This is caused by an increase in P_{CO_2} which reduces the HCO_3^-/P_{CO_2} ratio and thus depresses the pH. This corresponds to a movement from A to B in Figure 6-8. Whenever the P_{CO_2} rises, the bicarbonate must also increase to some extent because of dissociation of the carbonic acid produced. This is reflected by the left upward slope of the blood buffer line in Figure 6-8. However, the ratio HCO_3^-/P_{CO_2} falls. CO_2 retention can be caused by hypoventilation or ventilation-perfusion inequality.

If respiratory acidosis persists, the kidney responds by conserving HCO_3^-. It is prompted to do this by the increased P_{CO_2} in the renal tubular cells, which then excrete a more acid urine by secreting H^+ ions. The H^+ ions are excreted as $H_2PO_4^-$ or NH_4^+; the HCO_3^- ions are reabsorbed. The resulting increase in plasma HCO_3^- then moves the HCO_3^-/P_{CO_2} ratio back up toward its normal level. This corresponds to the movement from B to D along the line $P_{CO_2} = 60$ mm Hg in Figure 6-8 and is known as *compensated respiratory acidosis*. Typical events would be

$$pH = 6.1 + \log \frac{24}{0.03 \times 40} = 6.1 + \log 20 = 7.4 \qquad \text{(Normal)}$$

$$pH = 6.1 + \log \frac{28}{0.03 \times 60} = 6.1 + \log 15.6 = 7.29$$
$$\text{(Respiratory acidosis)}$$

$$pH = 6.1 + \log \frac{33}{0.03 \times 60} = 6.1 + \log 18.3 = 7.36$$
$$\text{(Compensated respiratory acidosis)}$$

The renal compensation is typically not complete, and so the pH does not fully return to its normal level of 7.4. The extent of the renal compensation can be determined from the *base excess*, that is, the vertical distance between the buffer lines BA and DE.

Respiratory Alkalosis

This is caused by a decrease in P_{CO_2}, which increases the HCO_3^-/P_{CO_2} ratio and thus elevates the pH (movement from A to C in Figure 6-8). A decrease in P_{CO_2} is caused by hyperventilation, for example, at high altitude (see Chapter 9). Renal compensation occurs by an increased excretion of bicarbonate, thus returning the HCO_3^-/P_{CO_2} ratio back toward normal (C to F along the line P_{CO_2} = 20 mm Hg). After a prolonged stay at high altitude, the renal compensation may be nearly complete. There is a negative base excess, or a *base deficit*.

Metabolic Acidosis

In this context, "metabolic" means a primary change in HCO_3^-, that is, the numerator of the Henderson-Hasselbalch equation. In metabolic acidosis, the ratio of HCO_3^- to P_{CO_2} falls, thus depressing the pH. The HCO_3^- may be lowered by the accumulation of acids in the blood, as in uncontrolled diabetes mellitus, or after tissue hypoxia, which releases lactic acid. The corresponding change in Figure 6-8 is a movement from A toward G.

In this instance, respiratory compensation occurs by an increase in ventilation that lowers the P_{CO_2} and raises the depressed HCO_3^-/P_{CO_2} ratio. The stimulus to raise the ventilation is chiefly the action of H^+ ions on the peripheral chemoreceptors (Chapter 8). In Figure 6-8, the point moves in the direction G to F (although not as far as F). There is a base deficit or negative base excess.

Metabolic Alkalosis

Here an increase in HCO_3^- raises the HCO_3^-/P_{CO_2} ratio and, thus, the pH. Excessive ingestion of alkalis and loss of acid gastric secretion by vomiting are causes. In Figure 6-8, the movement is in the direction A to E. Some respiratory compensation sometimes occurs by a reduction in alveolar ventilation that raises the P_{CO_2}. Point E then moves in the direction of D (although not all the way). However, respiratory compensation in metabolic alkalosis is often small and may be absent. Base excess is increased.

Note that mixed respiratory and metabolic disturbances often occur, and it may then be difficult to unravel the sequence of events.

Four Types of Acid-Base Disturbances

$$pH = pK + \log \frac{HCO_3^-}{0.03\ P_{CO_2}}$$

	Primary	Compensation
Acidosis		
Respiratory	$P_{CO_2} \uparrow$	$HCO_3^- \uparrow$
Metabolic	$HCO_3^- \downarrow$	$P_{CO_2} \downarrow$
Alkalosis		
Respiratory	$P_{CO_2} \downarrow$	$HCO_3^- \downarrow$
Metabolic	$HCO_3^- \uparrow$	often none

Blood-Tissue Gas Exchange

O_2 and CO_2 move between the systemic capillary blood and the tissue cells by simple diffusion, just as they move between the capillary blood and alveolar gas in the lung. We saw in Chapter 3 that the rate of transfer of gas through a tissue sheet is proportional to the tissue area and the difference in gas partial pressure between the two sides, and inversely proportional to the thickness. The thickness of the blood-gas barrier is less than 0.5 μm, but the distance between open capillaries in resting muscle is on the order of 50 μm. During exercise, when the O_2 consumption of the muscle increases, additional capillaries open up, thus reducing the diffusion distance and increasing the area for diffusion. Because CO_2 diffuses about 20 times faster than O_2 through tissue (Figure 3-1), elimination of CO_2 is much less of a problem than is O_2 delivery.

The way in which the P_{O_2} falls in tissue between adjacent open capillaries is shown schematically in Figure 6-9. As the O_2 diffuses away from the capillary, it is consumed by tissue, and the P_{O_2} falls. In A, the balance between O_2 consumption and delivery (determined by the capillary P_{O_2} and the intercapillary distance) results in an adequate P_{O_2} in all the tissue. In B, the intercapillary distance or the O_2 consumption has been increased until the P_{O_2} at one point in the tissue falls to zero. This is referred to as a *critical* situation. In C, there is an anoxic region where aerobic (that is, O_2 utilizing) metabolism is impossible. Under these conditions, the tissue turns to anaerobic glycolysis with the formation of lactic acid.

There is evidence that much of the fall of P_{O_2} in peripheral tissues occurs in the immediate vicinity of the capillary wall and that the P_{O_2} in muscle cells, for example, is very low (1 to 3 mm Hg) and nearly uniform. This pattern can be explained by the presence of myoglobin in the cell that acts as a reservoir for O_2 and enhances its diffusion within the cell.

How low can the tissue P_{O_2} fall before O_2 utilization ceases? In measurements on suspensions of liver mitochondria *in vitro*, O_2 consumption continues at the same rate until the P_{O_2} falls to the region of 3 mm Hg. Thus, it appears that the purpose of the much higher P_{O_2} in capillary blood is to ensure an adequate pressure for diffusion of O_2 to the mitochondria and that at the sites of O_2 utilization the P_{O_2} may be very low.

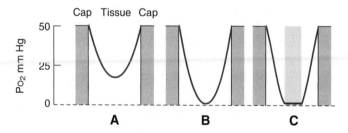

Figure 6-9. Scheme showing the fall of P_{O_2} between adjacent open capillaries. In **A**, oxygen delivery is adequate; in **B**, critical; and in **C**, inadequate for aerobic metabolism in the central core of tissue.

An abnormally low P_{O_2} in tissues is called tissue hypoxia. This is frequently caused by low O_2 delivery, which can be expressed as the cardiac output multiplied by the arterial O_2 concentration, or $\dot{Q} \times Ca_{O_2}$. The factors that determine Ca_{O_2} were discussed on page 65. Tissue hypoxia can be due to (1) a low P_{O_2} in arterial blood caused, for example, by pulmonary disease ("hypoxic hypoxia"); (2) a reduced ability of blood to carry O_2 as in anemia or carbon monoxide poisoning ("anemic hypoxia"); or (3) a reduction in tissue blood flow, either generalized, as in shock, or because of local obstruction ("circulatory hypoxia"). A fourth cause is some toxic substance that interferes with the ability of the tissues to utilize available O_2 ("histotoxic hypoxia"). An example is cyanide, which prevents the use of O_2 by cytochrome oxidase. In this case, the O_2 concentration of venous blood is high, and the O_2 consumption of the tissue extremely low because these are related by the Fick principle as applied to peripheral O_2 consumption. Table 6-1 summarizes some of the features of the different types of hypoxemia and tissue hypoxia.

Table 6-1. Features of Different Types of Hypoxemia or Tissue Hypoxia[a]

	P_{AO_2}	P_{ACO_2}	P_{aO_2}	P_{aCO_2}	C_{aO_2}	S_{aO_2}	$P_{\bar{v}O_2}$	$C_{\bar{v}O_2}$	O_2 Administration Helpful?
Lungs									
Hypoventilation	↓	↑	—	↑	—	—	—	—	Yes
Diffusion impairment	O	O	—	O	—	—	—	—	Yes
Shunt	O	O	—	O	—	—	—	—	Yes[b]
$\dot{V}_A/\dot{Q}$ inequality	Varies	↑ or O	—	↑ or O	—	—	—	—	Yes
Blood									
Anemia	O	O	O	O	—	O	—	—	Yes[b]
CO poisoning	O	O	O	O	—	O[c]	—	—	Yes[b]
Tissue									
Cyanide poisoning	O	O	O	O	O	O	↑	↑	No

[a] O, normal; ↑ increased; ↓ decreased.
[b] Of some (but limited) value because of increased dissolved oxygen.
[c] If O_2 saturation is calculated for hemoglobin not bound to CO.

QUESTIONS

For each question, choose the one best answer.

1. The presence of hemoglobin in normal arterial blood increases its oxygen concentration approximately how many times?
   A. 10
   B. 30
   C. 50
   D. 70
   E. 90

2. An increase in which of the following increases the O_2 affinity of hemoglobin?
   A. Temperature.
   B. P_{CO_2}.
   C. H^+ concentration.
   D. 2,3 DPG.
   E. Carbon monoxide added to the blood.

3. A patient with carbon monoxide poisoning is treated with hyperbaric oxygen that increases the arterial P_{O_2} to 2,000 mm Hg. The amount of oxygen dissolved in the arterial blood (in ml · 100 ml^{-1}) is:
   A. 2
   B. 3
   C. 4
   D. 5
   E. 6

4. A patient with severe anemia has normal lungs. Which of the following is most likely to be **FALSE**?
   A. Normal arterial P_{O_2}.
   B. Normal arterial O_2 saturation.
   C. Low arterial O_2 concentration.
   D. Low oxygen concentration of mixed venous blood.
   E. Normal tissue P_{O_2}.

5. All of the following statements are true about acute carbon monoxide poisoning **EXCEPT**:
   A. Reduced arterial P_{O_2}.
   B. Reduced oxygen concentration of arterial blood.
   C. Reduced oxygen concentration of mixed venous blood.
   D. O_2 dissociation curve is shifted to the left.
   E. Carbon monoxide is colorless and odorless.

6. The laboratory reports the following arterial blood gas values in a patient with severe lung disease who is breathing air: P_{O_2} 60 mm Hg, P_{CO_2} 110 mm Hg, pH 7.20. All of the following statements are true **EXCEPT**:
   A. Patient has hypoxemia.
   B. Patient has severe CO_2 retention.
   C. There is a respiratory acidosis.
   D. The respiratory acidosis is partially compensated.
   E. The values for P_{O_2} and P_{CO_2} are internally consistent.

7. Most of the carbon dioxide transported in the blood is in the form of:
   A. Dissolved.
   B. Bicarbonate.
   C. Attached to hemoglobin.
   D. As carbamino compounds.
   E. Carbonic acid.

8. A patient with chronic lung disease has arterial P_{O_2} and P_{CO_2} values of 50 and 60 mm Hg, respectively, and a pH of 7.35. How is his acid-base status best described?
   A. Normal.
   B. Partially compensated respiratory alkalosis.
   C. Partially compensated respiratory acidosis.
   D. Metabolic acidosis.
   E. Metabolic alkalosis.

9. The P_{O_2} (in mm Hg) inside skeletal muscle cells during exercise is closest to:
   A. 3
   B. 10
   C. 20
   D. 30
   E. 40

10. A patient with chronic pulmonary disease undergoes emergency surgery. Postoperatively the arterial P_{O_2}, P_{CO_2} and pH are 50 mm Hg, 50 mm Hg and 7.20, respectively. How would the acid-base status be best described?
   A. Mixed respiratory and metabolic acidosis.
   B. Uncompensated respiratory acidosis.
   C. Fully compensated respiratory acidosis.
   D. Uncompensated metabolic acidosis.
   E. Fully compensated metabolic acidosis.

11. The laboratory provides the following report on arterial blood from a patient: P_{CO_2} 32 mm Hg, pH 7.25, HCO^-_3 concentration 25 mmol $\cdot$ l^{-1}. You conclude that there is:
   A. Respiratory alkalosis with metabolic compensation.
   B. Acute respiratory acidosis.
   C. Metabolic acidosis with respiratory compensation.
   D. Metabolic alkalosis with respiratory compensation.
   E. A laboratory error.

12. A patient with shortness of breath is breathing air at sea level and an arterial blood sample shows P_{O_2} 90 mm Hg, P_{CO_2} 32 mm Hg, pH 7.30. Assuming that the respiratory exchange ratio is 0.8, these data indicate:
   A. Primary respiratory alkalosis with metabolic compensation.
   B. Normal alveolar-arterial P_{O_2} difference.
   C. Arterial O_2 saturation < 70%.
   D. The sample was mistakenly taken from a vein.
   E. Partially compensated metabolic acidosis.

Mechanics of Breathing
How the Lung Is Supported and Moved

We saw in Chapter 2 that gas gets to and from the alveoli by the process of ventilation. We now turn to the forces that move the lung and chest wall, and the resistances that they overcome. First we consider the muscles of respiration, both inspiration and expiration. Then we look at the factors determining the elastic properties of the lung including the tissue elements and the air-liquid surface tension. Next we examine the mechanism of regional differences in ventilation and also the closure of small airways. Just as the lung is elastic so is the chest wall and we look at the interaction between the two. The physical

principles of airway resistance are then considered along with its measurement, chief site in the lung, and physiological factors that affect it. Dynamic
compression of the airways during a forced expiration is analyzed. Finally the
work required to move the lung and chest wall is considered.

Muscles of Respiration

Inspiration

The most important muscle of inspiration is the *diaphragm*. This consists of a thin,
dome-shaped sheet of muscle that is inserted into the lower ribs. It is supplied by
the phrenic nerves from cervical segments 3, 4, and 5. When it contracts, the abdominal contents are forced downward and forward, and the vertical dimension
of the chest cavity is increased. In addition, the rib margins are lifted and moved
out, causing an increase in the transverse diameter of the thorax (Figure 7-1).

In normal tidal breathing, the level of the diaphragm moves about 1 cm or so,
but on forced inspiration and expiration, a total excursion of up to 10 cm may occur. When the diaphragm is paralyzed, it moves *up* rather than *down* with inspiration because the intrathoracic pressure falls. This is known as *paradoxical movement* and can be demonstrated at fluoroscopy when the subject sniffs.

The *external intercostal muscles* connect adjacent ribs and slope downward and
forward (Figure 7-2). When they contract, the ribs are pulled upward and forward,
causing an increase in both the lateral and anteroposterior diameters of the thorax. The lateral dimension increases because of the "bucket-handle" movement
of the ribs. The intercostal muscles are supplied by intercostal nerves that come
off the spinal cord at the same level. Paralysis of the intercostal muscles alone
does not seriously affect breathing because the diaphragm is so effective.

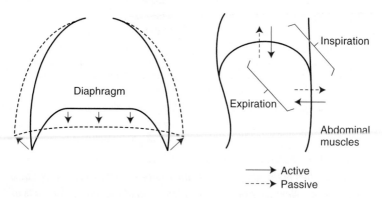

Figure 7-1. On inspiration, the dome-shaped diaphragm contracts, the abdominal
contents are forced down and forward, and the rib cage is widened. Both increase
the volume of the thorax. On forced expiration, the abdominal muscles contract
and push the diaphragm up.

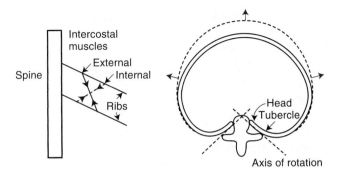

Figure 7-2. When the external intercostal muscles contract, the ribs are pulled upward and forward, and they rotate on an axis joining the tubercle and head of rib. As a result, both the lateral and anteroposterior diameters of the thorax increase. The internal intercostals have the opposite action.

The *accessory muscles of inspiration* include the scalene muscles which elevate the first two ribs, and the sternomastoids which raise the sternum. There is little, if any, activity in these muscles during quiet breathing, but during exercise they may contract vigorously. Other muscles that play a minor role include the alae nasi, which cause flaring of the nostrils, and small muscles in the neck and head.

Expiration

This is passive during quiet breathing. The lung and chest wall are elastic and tend to return to their equilibrium positions after being actively expanded during inspiration. During exercise and voluntary hyperventilation, expiration becomes active. The most important muscles of expiration are those of the *abdominal wall*, including the rectus abdominis, internal and external oblique muscles, and transversus abdominis. When these muscles contract, intra-abdominal pressure is raised, and the diaphragm is pushed upward. These muscles also contract forcefully during coughing, vomiting, and defecation.

The *internal intercostal muscles* assist active expiration by pulling the ribs downward and inward (opposite to the action of the external intercostal muscles), thus decreasing the thoracic volume. In addition, they stiffen the intercostal spaces to prevent them from bulging outward during straining. Experimental studies show that the actions of the respiratory muscles, especially the intercostals, are more complicated than this brief account suggests.

Respiratory Muscles

- Inspiration is active; expiration is passive during rest
- Diaphragm is the most important muscle of inspiration; it is supplied by phrenic nerves which originate high in the cervical region
- Other muscles include the intercostals, abdominal muscles, and accessory muscles

Elastic Properties of the Lung

Pressure-Volume Curve

Suppose we take an excised animal lung, cannulate the trachea, and place it in-side a jar (Figure 7-3). When the pressure within the jar is reduced below atmo-spheric pressure, the lung expands and its change in volume can be measured with a spirometer. The pressure is held at each level, as indicated by the points, for a few seconds to allow the lung to come to rest. In this way, the pressure-volume curve of the lung can be plotted.

In Figure 7-3, the expanding pressure around the lung is generated by a pump, but in humans it is developed by an increase in volume of the chest cage. The fact that the intrapleural space between the lung and chest wall is much smaller than the space between the lung and the bottle in Figure 7-3 makes no essential dif-ference. The intrapleural space contains only a few milliliters of fluid.

Figure 7-3 shows that the curves which the lung follows during inflation and deflation are different. This behavior is known as *hysteresis*. Note that the lung volume at any given pressure during deflation is larger than during inflation. Note also that the lung without any expanding pressure has some air inside it. In fact, even if the pressure around the lung is raised above atmospheric pressure, little further air is lost because small airways close, trapping gas in the alveoli (compare Figure 7-9). This *airway closure* occurs at higher lung volumes with increasing age and also in some types of lung disease.

In Figure 7-3 the pressure inside the airways and alveoli of the lung is the same as atmospheric pressure, which is zero on the horizontal axis. Thus, this axis also measures the difference in pressure between the inside and outside of the lung. This is known as *transpulmonary pressure* and is numerically equal to the pressure

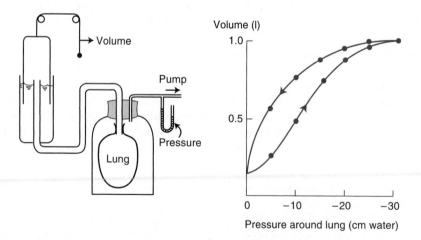

Figure 7-3. Measurement of the pressure-volume curve of excised lung. The lung is held at each pressure for a few seconds while its volume is measured. The curve is nonlinear and becomes flatter at high expanding pressures. Note that the infla-tion and deflation curves are not the same; this is called hysteresis.

around the lung when the alveolar pressure is atmospheric. It is also possible to measure the pressure-volume relationship of the lung shown in Figure 7-3 by inflating it with positive pressure and leaving the pleural surface exposed to the atmosphere. In this case, the horizontal axis could be labeled "airway pressure," and the values would be positive. The curves would be identical to those shown in Figure 7-3.

Compliance

The slope of the pressure-volume curve, or the volume change per unit pressure change, is known as the *compliance*. In the normal range (expanding pressure of about −5 to −10 cm water) the lung is remarkably distensible or very compliant. The compliance of the human lung is about 200 ml · cm water^{-1}. However, at high expanding pressures, the lung is stiffer, and its compliance is smaller, as shown by the flatter slope of the curve.

A *reduced* compliance is caused by an increase of fibrous tissue in the lung (pulmonary fibrosis). In addition, compliance is reduced by alveolar edema which prevents the inflation of some alveoli. Compliance also falls if the lung remains unventilated for a long period, especially if its volume is low. This may be partly caused by atelectasis (collapse) of some units, but increases in surface tension also occur (see below). Compliance is also reduced somewhat if the pulmonary venous pressure is increased and the lung becomes engorged with blood.

An *increased* compliance occurs in pulmonary emphysema and in the normal aging lung. In both instances, an alteration in the elastic tissue in the lung is probably responsible. Increased compliance also occurs during an asthma attack, but the reason is unclear.

The compliance of lung depends on its size. Clearly, the change in volume per unit change of pressure will be larger for a human lung than, say, a mouse lung. For this reason, the compliance per unit volume of lung, or *specific compliance*, is sometimes measured if we wish to draw conclusions about the intrinsic elastic properties of the lung tissue.

The pressure surrounding the lung is less than atmospheric in Figure 7-3 (and in the living chest) because of the elastic recoil of the lung. What is responsible for the lung's elastic behavior, that is, its tendency to return to its resting volume after distension? One factor is the elastic tissue which is visible in histological sections. Fibers of elastin and collagen can be seen in the alveolar walls and around vessels and bronchi. Probably the elastic behavior of the lung has less to do with simple elongation of these fibers than it does with their geometrical arrangement. An analogy is a nylon stocking which is very distensible because of its knitted make-up, although the individual nylon fibers are very difficult to stretch. The changes in elastic recoil that occur in the lung with age and in emphysema are presumably caused by changes in this elastic tissue.

Surface Tension

Another important factor in the pressure-volume behavior of lung is the surface tension of the liquid film lining the alveoli. Surface tension is the force (in dynes, for example) acting across an imaginary line 1-cm long in the surface of the liquid (Figure 7-4A). It arises because the attractive forces between adjacent molecules of the liquid are much stronger than those between the liquid and gas, with the result that the liquid surface area becomes as small as possible. This behavior is seen clearly in a soap bubble blown on the end of a tube (Figure 7-4B). The surfaces of the bubble contract as much as they can, forming a sphere (smallest surface area for a given volume) and generating a pressure that can be predicted from Laplace's law: pressure = (4 × surface tension)/radius. When only one surface is involved in a liquid-lined spherical alveolus, the numerator has the number 2 rather than 4.

The first evidence that surface tension might contribute to the pressure-volume behavior of the lung was obtained by early physiologists when they showed that lungs inflated with saline have a much larger compliance (are easier to distend) than air-filled lungs (Figure 7-5). Because the saline abolished the surface tension forces but presumably did not affect the tissue forces of the lung, this observation meant that surface tension contributed a large part of the static recoil force of the lung. Some time later, workers studying edema foam coming from the lungs of animals exposed to noxious gases noticed that the tiny air bubbles of the foam were extremely stable. They recognized that this indicated a very low surface tension, an observation which led to the remarkable discovery of pulmonary *surfactant*.

Figure 7-4. A. Surface tension is the force (in dynes, for example) acting across an imaginary line 1 cm long in a liquid surface. **B.** Surface forces in a soap bubble tend to reduce the area of the surface and generate a pressure within the bubble. **C.** Because the smaller bubble generates a larger pressure, it blows up the larger bubble.

Figure 7-5. Comparison of pressure-volume curves of air-filled and saline-filled lungs (cat). *Open circles,* inflation; *closed circles,* deflation. Note that the saline-filled lung has a higher compliance and also much less hysteresis than the air-filled lung.

It is now known that some of the cells lining the alveoli secrete a material that profoundly lowers the surface tension of the alveolar lining fluid. Surfactant is a phospholipid, and dipalmitoyl phosphatidylcholine (DPPC) is an important constituent. Alveolar epithelial cells are of two types. Type I cells have the shape of a fried egg with long cytoplasmic extensions spreading out thinly over the alveolar walls (Figure 1-1). Type II cells are more compact (Figure 7-6), and electron microscopy shows lamellated bodies within them that are extruded into the alveoli and transform into surfactant. Some of the surfactant can be washed out of animal lungs by rinsing them with saline.

The phospholipid DPPC is synthesized in the lung from fatty acids that are either extracted from the blood or are themselves synthesized in the lung. Synthesis is fast, and there is a rapid turnover of surfactant. If the blood flow to a region of lung is abolished as the result of an embolus, for example, the surfactant there may be depleted. Surfactant is formed relatively late in fetal life, and babies born without adequate amounts develop respiratory distress and may die.

The effects of this material on surface tension can be studied with a surface balance (Figure 7-7). This consists of a tray containing saline on which a small amount of test material is placed. The area of the surface is then alternately expanded and compressed by a movable barrier while the surface tension is measured from the force exerted on a platinum strip. Pure saline gives a surface tension of about 70 dynes/cm, regardless of the area of its surface. Adding detergent reduces the surface tension, but again this is independent of area. When lung washings are placed on the saline, the curve shown in Figure 7-7B is obtained. Note that the surface tension changes greatly with the surface area and that there

Figure 7-6. Electron micrograph of type II epithelial cell (×10,000). Note the lamellated bodies (LB), large nucleus, and microvilli (*arrows*). The *inset at top right* is a scanning electron micrograph showing the surface view of a type II cell with its characteristic distribution of microvilli (×3400).

is hysteresis (compare Figure 7-3). Note also that the surface tension falls to extremely low values when the area is small.

How does surfactant reduce the surface tension so much? Apparently the molecules of DPPC are hydrophobic at one end and hydrophilic at the other, and they align themselves in the surface. When this occurs, their intermolecular repulsive forces oppose the normal attracting forces between the liquid surface molecules that are responsible for surface tension. The reduction in surface tension is greater when the film is compressed because the molecules of DPPC are then crowded closer together and repel each other more.

What are the physiological advantages of surfactant? First, a low surface tension in the alveoli increases the compliance of the lung and reduces the work of expanding it with each breath. Next, stability of the alveoli is promoted. The 300 million alveoli appear to be inherently unstable because areas of atelectasis (collapse) often form in the presence of disease. This is a complex subject, but one way of looking at the lung is to regard it as a collection of millions of tiny bubbles (although this is clearly an oversimplification). In such an arrangement, there is

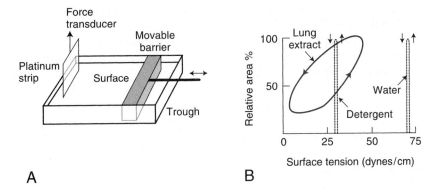

Figure 7-7. A. Surface balance. The area of the surface is altered, and the surface tension is measured from the force exerted on a platinum strip dipped into the surface. **B.** Plots of surface tension and area obtained with a surface balance. Note that lung washings show a change in surface tension with area and that the minimal tension is very small. The axes are chosen to allow a comparison with the pressure-volume curve of the lung (Figures 7-3 and 7-5).

a tendency for small bubbles to collapse and blow up large ones. Figure 7-4C shows that the pressure generated by the surface forces in a bubble is inversely proportional to its radius, with the result that if the surface tensions are the same, the pressure inside a small bubble exceeds that in a large bubble. However, Figure 7-7 shows that when lung washings are present, a small surface area is associated with a small surface tension. Thus, the tendency for small alveoli to empty into large alveoli is apparently reduced.

A third role of surfactant is to help to keep the alveoli dry. Just as the surface tension forces tend to collapse alveoli, they also tend to suck fluid into the alveolar spaces from the capillaries. In effect, the surface tension of the curved alveolar surface reduces the hydrostatic pressure in the tissue outside the capillaries. By reducing these surface forces, surfactant prevents the transudation of fluid.

What are the consequences of loss of surfactant? On the basis of its functions discussed above, we would expect these to be stiff lungs (low compliance), areas of atelectasis, and alveoli filled with transudate. Indeed, these are the pathophysiological features of the "infant respiratory distress syndrome," and this disease is caused by an absence of this crucial material. It is now possible to treat these infants by instilling synthesized surfactant into the lung.

Pulmonary Surfactant

- Reduces the surface tension of the alveolar lining layer
- Produced by type II alveolar epithelial cells
- Contains dipalmitoyl phosphatidylcholine
- Absence results in reduced lung compliance, alveolar atelectasis, and tendency to pulmonary edema

There is another mechanism that apparently contributes to the stability of the alveoli in the lung. Figures 1-2, 1-7, and 4-3 remind us that all the alveoli (except those immediately adjacent to the pleural surface) are surrounded by other alveoli and are therefore supported by each other. In a structure such as this with many connecting links, any tendency for one group of units to reduce or increase its volume relative to the rest of the structure is opposed. For example, if a group of alveoli has a tendency to collapse, large expanding forces will be developed on them because the surrounding parenchyma is expanded.

This support offered to lung units by those surrounding them is termed "interdependence." The same factors explain the development of low pressures around large blood vessels and airways as the lung expands (Figure 4-2).

Cause of Regional Differences in Ventilation

We saw in Figure 2-7 that the lower regions of the lung ventilate more than do the upper zones, and this is a convenient place to discuss the cause of these topographical differences. It has been shown that the intrapleural pressure is less negative at the bottom than the top of the lung (Figure 7-8). The reason for this is the weight of the lung. Anything that is supported requires a larger pressure below it than above it to balance the downward-acting weight forces, and the lung, which is partly supported by the rib cage and diaphragm, is no exception. Thus, the pressure near the base is higher (less negative) than at the apex.

Figure 7-8. Explanation of the regional differences of ventilation down the lung. Because of the weight of the lung, the intrapleural pressure is less negative at the base than at the apex. As a consequence, the basal lung is relatively compressed in its resting state but expands more on inspiration than the apex.

Figure 7-8 shows the way in which the volume of a portion of lung (for example, a lobe) expands as the pressure around it is decreased (compare Figure 7-1). The pressure inside the lung is the same as atmospheric pressure. Note that the lung is easier to inflate at low volumes than at high volumes, where it becomes stiffer. Because the expanding pressure at the base of the lung is small, this region has a small resting volume. However, because it is situated on a steep part of the pressure-volume curve, it expands well on inspiration. By contrast, the apex of the lung has a large expanding pressure, a big resting volume, and small change in volume in inspiration.*

Now when we talk of regional differences in ventilation, we mean the change in volume per unit resting volume. It is clear from Figure 7-8 that the base of the lung has both a larger change in volume and smaller resting volume than the apex. Thus, its ventilation is greater. Note the paradox that, although the base of the lung is relatively poorly expanded compared with the apex, it is better ventilated. The same explanation can be given for the large ventilation of dependent lung in both the supine and lateral positions.

A remarkable change in the distribution of ventilation occurs at low lung volumes. Figure 7-9 is similar to Figure 7-8 except that it represents the situation at

Figure 7-9. Situation at very low lung volumes. Now intrapleural pressures are less negative, and the pressure at the base actually exceeds airway (atmospheric) pressure. As a consequence, airway closure occurs in this region, and no gas enters with small inspirations.

* This explanation is an oversimplification because the pressure-volume behavior of a portion of a structure like the lung may not be identical to that of the whole organ.

residual volume (that is, after a full expiration, see Figure 2-2). Now the intrapleural pressures are less negative because the lung is not so well expanded and the elastic recoil forces are smaller. However, the differences between apex and base are still present because of the weight of the lung. Note that the intrapleural pressure at the base now actually exceeds airway (atmospheric) pressure. Under these conditions, the lung at the base is not being expanded but compressed, and ventilation is impossible until the local intrapleural pressure falls below atmospheric pressure. By contrast, the apex of the lung is on a favorable part of the pressure-volume curve and ventilates well. Thus, the normal distribution of ventilation is inverted, the upper regions ventilating better than the lower zones.

Airway Closure

The compressed region of lung at the base does not have all its gas squeezed out. In practice, small airways, probably in the region of respiratory bronchioles (Figure 1-4), close first, thus trapping gas in the distal alveoli. This *airway closure* occurs only at very low lung volumes in young normal subjects. However, in elderly apparently normal people, airway closure in the lowermost regions of the lung occurs at higher volumes and may be present at functional residual capacity (Figure 2-2). The reason for this is that the aging lung loses some of its elastic recoil, and intrapleural pressures therefore become less negative, thus approaching the situation shown in Figure 7-9. In these circumstances, dependent (that is, lowermost) regions of the lung may be only intermittently ventilated, and this leads to defective gas exchange (Chapter 5). A similar situation frequently develops in patients with some types of chronic lung disease.

Elastic Properties of the Chest Wall

Just as the lung is elastic, so is the thoracic cage. This can be illustrated by putting air into the intrapleural space (pneumothorax). Figure 7-10 shows that the normal pressure outside the lung is subatmospheric just as it is in the jar of Figure 7-3. When air is introduced into the intrapleural space, raising the pressure to atmospheric, the lung collapses inward, and the chest wall springs outward. This

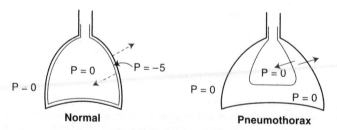

Figure 7-10. The tendency of the lung to recoil to its deflated volume is balanced by the tendency of the chest cage to bow out. As a result, the intrapleural pressure is subatmospheric. Pneumothorax allows the lung to collapse and the thorax to spring out.

Figure 7-11. Relaxation pressure-volume curve of the lung and chest wall. The subject inspires (or expires) to a certain volume from the spirometer, the tap is closed, and the subject then relaxes his respiratory muscles. The curve for lung + chest wall can be explained by the addition of the individual lung and chest wall curves.

shows that under equilibrium conditions, the chest wall is pulled inward while the lung is pulled outward, the two pulls balancing each other.

These interactions can be seen more clearly if we plot a pressure-volume curve for the lung and chest wall (Figure 7-11). For this, the subject inspires or expires from a spirometer and then relaxes the respiratory muscles while the airway pressure is measured ("relaxation pressure"). Incidentally, this is difficult for an untrained subject. Figure 7-11 shows that at functional residual capacity (FRC), the relaxation pressure of the lung and chest wall is atmospheric. Indeed, FRC is the equilibrium volume when the elastic recoil of the lung is balanced by the normal tendency for the chest wall to spring out. At volumes above this, the pressure is positive, and at smaller volumes, the pressure is subatmospheric.

Figure 7-11 also shows the curve for the lung alone. This is similar to that shown in Figure 7-3, except that for clarity no hysteresis is indicated and the pressures are positive instead of negative. They are the pressures that would be found from the experiment of Figure 7-3 if, after the lung had reached a certain volume, the line to the spirometer were clamped, the jar opened to the atmosphere (so that the lung relaxed against the closed airway), and the airway pressure measured. Note that at zero pressure the lung is at its minimal volume, which is below residual volume (RV).

The third curve is for the chest wall only. We can imagine this being measured on a subject with a normal chest wall and no lung! Note that at FRC the relaxation pressure is negative. In other words, at this volume the chest cage is tending to spring out. It is not until the volume is increased to about 75% of the vital capacity that the relaxation pressure is atmospheric, that is, that the chest wall has found its equilibrium position. At every volume, the relaxation pressure of the lung plus chest wall is the sum of the pressures for the lung and the chest wall measured separately. Because the pressure (at a given volume) is inversely proportional to compliance, this implies that the total compliance of the lung and chest wall is the sum of the reciprocals of the lung and chest wall compliances measured separately, or $1/C_T = 1/C_L + 1/C_{CW}$.

Relaxation Pressure-Volume Curve

- Elastic properties of both the lung and chest wall determine their combined volume
- At FRC, the inward pull of the lung is balanced by the outward spring of the chest wall
- Lung retracts at all volumes above minimal volume
- Chest wall tends to expand at volumes up to about 75% of vital capacity

---

Airway Resistance

Airflow Through Tubes

If air flows through a tube (Figure 7-12), a difference of pressure exists between the ends. The pressure difference depends on the rate and pattern of flow. At low flow rates, the stream lines are parallel to the sides of the tube (A). This is known as laminar flow. As the flow rate is increased, unsteadiness develops, especially at branches. Here, separation of the stream lines from the wall may occur with the formation of local eddies (B). At still higher flow rates, complete disorganization of the stream lines is seen; this is turbulence (C).

The pressure-flow characteristics for *laminar flow* were first described by the French physician Poiseuille. In straight circular tubes, the volume flow rate is given by

$$\dot{V} = \frac{P\pi r^4}{8nl}$$

where P is the driving pressure (ΔP in Figure 7-12A), r radius, n viscosity, and l length. It can be seen that driving pressure is proportional to flow rate, or $P = K\dot{V}$.

Figure 7-12. Patterns of airflow in tubes. In A, the flow is laminar; in B, transitional with eddy formation at branches; and in C, turbulent. Resistance is (P_1-P_2)/flow.

Because flow resistance R is driving pressure divided by flow (compare p. 32), we have

$$R = \frac{8nl}{\pi r^4}$$

Note the critical importance of tube radius; if the radius is halved, the resistance increases 16-fold! However, doubling the length only doubles resistance. Note also that the viscosity of the gas, but not its density, affects the pressure-flow relationship.

Another feature of laminar flow when it is fully developed is that the gas in the center of the tube moves twice as fast as the average velocity. Thus, a spike of rapidly moving gas travels down the axis of the tube (Figure 7-12A). This changing velocity across the diameter of the tube is known as the *velocity profile*.

Turbulent flow has different properties. Here pressure is not proportional to flow rate but, approximately, to its square: $P = K\dot{V}^2$. In addition, the viscosity of the gas becomes relatively unimportant, but an increase in gas density increases the pressure drop for a given flow. Turbulent flow does not have the high axial flow velocity that is characteristic of laminar flow.

Whether flow will be laminar or turbulent depends to a large extent on the Reynolds number, Re. This is given by

$$Re = \frac{2rvd}{n}$$

where d is density, v average velocity, r radius, and n viscosity. Because density and velocity are in the numerator, and viscosity is in the denominator, the expression gives the ratio of inertial to viscous forces. In straight, smooth tubes, turbulence is probable when the Reynolds number exceeds 2000. The expression shows that turbulence is most likely to occur when the velocity of flow is high and the tube diameter is large (for a given velocity). Note also that a low-density gas like helium tends to produce less turbulence.

In such a complicated system of tubes as the bronchial tree with its many branches, changes in caliber, and irregular wall surfaces, the application of the above principles is difficult. In practice, for laminar flow to occur, the entrance conditions of the tube are critical. If eddy formation occurs upstream at a branch point, this disturbance is carried downstream some distance before it disappears. Thus, in a rapidly branching system like the lung, fully developed laminar flow (Figure 7-12A) probably only occurs in the very small airways where the Reynolds numbers are very low (approximately 1 in terminal bronchioles). In most of the bronchial tree, flow is transitional (B), while true turbulence may occur in the trachea, especially on exercise when flow velocities are high. In general, driving pressure is determined by both the flow rate and its square: $P = K_1\dot{V} + K_2\dot{V}^2$.

Laminar and Turbulent Flow

- In laminar flow, resistance is determined by the fourth power of the radius
- In laminar flow, the velocity profile shows a central spike of fast gas
- Turbulent flow is most likely to occur at high Reynolds numbers, that is when inertial forces dominate over viscous forces

---

Measurement of Airway Resistance

Airway resistance is the pressure difference between the alveoli and the mouth divided by a flow rate (Figure 7-12). Mouth pressure is easily measured with a manometer. Alveolar pressure can be deduced from measurements made in a body plethysmograph. More information on this technique is given on p. 162.

Pressures During the Breathing Cycle

Suppose we measure the pressures in the intrapleural and alveolar spaces during normal breathing.[†] Figure 7-13 shows that before inspiration begins, the intrapleural pressure is −5 cm water because of the elastic recoil of the lung (compare Figures 7-3 and 7-10). Alveolar pressure is zero (atmospheric) because with no airflow, there is no pressure drop along the airways. However, for inspiratory flow to occur, the alveolar pressure falls, thus establishing the driving pressure (Figure 7-12). Indeed, the extent of the fall depends on the flow rate and the resistance of the airways. In normal subjects, the change in alveolar pressure is only 1-cm water or so, but in patients with airway obstruction, it may be many times that.

Intrapleural pressure falls during inspiration for two reasons. First, as the lung expands, its elastic recoil increases (Figure 7-3). This alone would cause the in-

---

[†] Intrapleural pressure can be estimated by placing a balloon catheter in the esophagus.

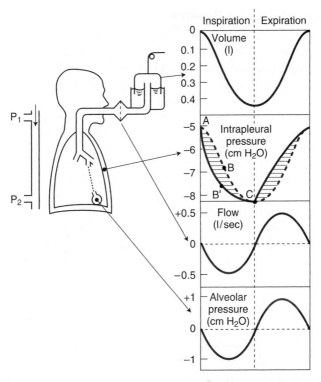

Figure 7-13. Pressures during the breathing cycle. If there were no airway resistance, alveolar pressure would remain at zero, and intrapleural pressure would follow the *broken line* ABC, which is determined by the elastic recoil of the lung. Airway (and tissue) resistance contributes the *hatched portion* of intrapleural pressure (see text).

trapleural pressure to move along the broken line ABC. In addition, however, the pressure drop along the airway is associated with a further fall in intrapleural pressure,[‡] represented by the hatched area, so that the actual path is AB'C. Thus, the vertical distance between lines ABC and AB'C reflects the alveolar pressure at any instant. As an equation of pressures, (mouth − intrapleural) = (mouth − alveolar) + (alveolar − intrapleural).

On expiration, similar changes occur. Now intrapleural pressure is *less* negative than it would be in the absence of airway resistance because alveolar pressure is positive. Indeed, with a forced expiration, intrapleural pressure goes above zero.

Note that the shape of the alveolar pressure tracing is similar to that of flow. Indeed, they would be identical if the airway resistance remained constant during the cycle. Also, the intrapleural pressure curve ABC would have the same shape as the volume tracing if the lung compliance remained constant.

[‡] There is also a contribution made by tissue resistance, which is considered later in this chapter.

Chief Site of Airway Resistance

As the airways penetrate toward the periphery of the lung, they become more numerous but much narrower (see Figures 1-3 and 1-5). Based on Poiseuille's equation with its (radius)^4 term, it would be natural to think that the major part of the resistance lies in the very narrow airways. Indeed, this was thought to be the case for many years. However, it has now been shown by direct measurements of the pressure drop along the bronchial tree that the major site of resistance is the medium-sized bronchi and that the very small bronchioles contribute relatively little resistance. Figure 7-14 shows that most of the pressure drop occurs in the airways up to the seventh generation. Less than 20% can be attributed to airways less than 2 mm in diameter (about generation 8). The reason for this apparent paradox is the prodigious number of small airways.

The fact that the peripheral airways contribute so little resistance is important in the detection of early airway disease. Because they constitute a "silent zone," it is probable that considerable small airway disease can be present before the usual measurements of airway resistance can detect an abnormality. This issue is considered in more detail in Chapter 10.

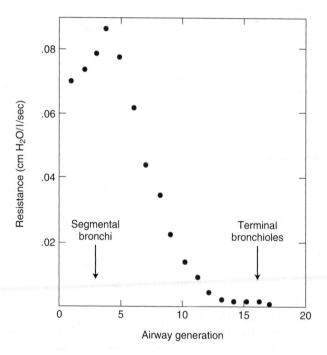

Figure 7-14. Location of the chief site of airway resistance. Note that the intermediate-sized bronchi contribute most of the resistance and that relatively little is located in the very small airways.

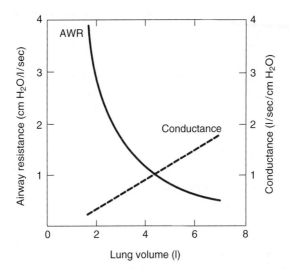

Figure 7-15. Variation of airway resistance (AWR) with lung volume. If the reciprocal of airway resistance (conductance) is plotted, the graph is a straight line.

Factors Determining Airway Resistance

Lung volume has an important effect on airway resistance. Like the extra-alveolar blood vessels (Figure 4-2), the bronchi are supported by the radial traction of the surrounding lung tissue, and their caliber is increased as the lung expands (compare Figure 4-6). Figure 7-15 shows that as lung volume is reduced, airway resistance rises rapidly. If the reciprocal of resistance (conductance) is plotted against lung volume, an approximately linear relationship is obtained.

At very low lung volumes, the small airways may close completely, especially at the bottom of the lung, where the lung is less well expanded (Figure 7-9). Patients who have increased airway resistance often breathe at high lung volumes; this helps to reduce their airway resistance.

Contraction of *bronchial smooth muscle* narrows the airways and increases airway resistance. This may occur reflexly through the stimulation of receptors in the trachea and large bronchi by irritants such as cigarette smoke. Motor innervation is by the vagus nerve. The tone of the smooth muscle is under the control of the autonomic nervous system. Stimulation of adrenergic receptors causes bronchodilatation as do epinephrine and isoproterenol.

β-Adrenergic receptors are of two types: β_1 receptors occur principally in the heart, while β_2 receptors relax smooth muscle in the bronchi, blood vessels, and uterus. Selective β_2-adrenergic agonists are now extensively used in the treatments of asthma.

Parasympathetic activity causes bronchoconstriction, as does acetylcholine. A fall of P_{CO_2} in alveolar gas causes an increase in airway resistance, apparently as a result of a direct action on bronchiolar smooth muscle. The injection of his-

---

Airway Resistance

- Highest in the medium-sized bronchi; low in very small airways
- Decreases as lung volume rises because the airways are then pulled open
- Bronchial smooth muscle is controlled by the autonomic nervous system; stimulation of β-adrenergic receptors causes bronchodilatation
- Breathing a dense gas as in diving increases resistance

---

tamine into the pulmonary artery causes constriction of smooth muscle located in the alveolar ducts.

The *density* and *viscosity* of the inspired gas affect the resistance offered to flow. The resistance is increased during a deep dive because the increased pressure raises gas density, but it is reduced when a helium-O_2 mixture is breathed. The fact that changes in density rather than viscosity have such an influence on resistance is evidence that flow is not purely laminar in the medium-sized airways, where the main site of resistance lies (Figure 7-14).

Dynamic Compression of Airways

Suppose a subject inspires to total lung capacity and then exhales as hard as possible to residual volume. We can record a *flow-volume curve* like A in Figure 7-16, which shows that flow rises very rapidly to a high value but then declines over most of expiration. A remarkable feature of this flow-volume envelope is that it is virtually impossible to penetrate it. For example, no matter whether we start exhaling slowly and then accelerate, as in B, or make a less forceful expiration, as in C, the descending portion of the flow-volume curve takes virtually the same path.

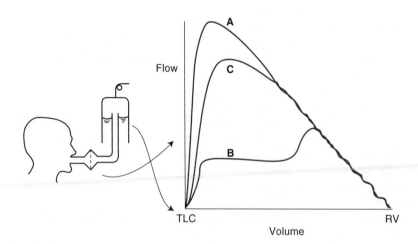

Figure 7-16. Flow-volume curves. In *A*, a maximal inspiration was followed by a forced expiration. In *B*, expiration was initially slow and then forced. In *C*, expiratory effort was submaximal. In all three, the descending portions of the curves are almost superimposed.

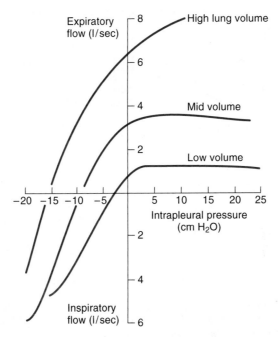

Figure 7-17. Isovolume pressure-flow curves drawn for three lung volumes. Each of these was obtained from a series of forced expirations and inspirations (see text). Note that at the high lung volume, a rise in intrapleural pressure (obtained by increasing expiratory effort) results in a greater expiratory flow. However, at mid and low volumes, flow becomes independent of effort after a certain intrapleural pressure has been exceeded.

Thus, something powerful is limiting expiratory flow, and over most of the lung volume, flow rate is independent of effort.

We can get more information about this curious state of affairs by plotting the data in another way, as shown in Figure 7-17. For this, the subject takes a series of maximal inspirations (or expirations) and then exhales (or inhales) fully with varying degrees of effort. If the flow rates and intrapleural pressures are plotted at the *same* lung volume for each expiration and inspiration, so-called *isovolume pressure-flow curves* can be obtained. It can be seen that at high lung volumes, the expiratory flow rate continues to increase with effort, as might be expected. However, at mid or low volumes, the flow rate reaches a plateau and cannot be increased with further increase in intrapleural pressure. Under these conditions, flow is therefore *effort independent.*

The reason for this remarkable behavior is compression of the airways by intrathoracic pressure. Figure 7-18 shows schematically the forces acting across an airway within the lung. The pressure outside the airway is shown as intrapleural, although this is an oversimplification. In A, before inspiration has begun, airway pressure is everywhere zero (no flow), and because intrapleural pressure is −5 cm water, there is a pressure of 5 cm water holding the airway open. As inspiration

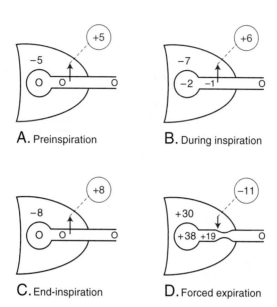

A. Preinspiration   B. During inspiration

C. End-inspiration   D. Forced expiration

Figure 7-18. Scheme showing why airways are compressed during forced expiration. Note that the pressure difference across the airway is holding it open, except during a forced expiration. See text for details.

starts (B), both intrapleural and alveolar pressure fall by 2 cm water (same lung volume as A and tissue resistance is neglected), and flow begins. Because of the pressure drop along the airway, the pressure inside is −1 cm water, and there is a pressure of 6 cm water holding the airway open. At end-inspiration (C), again flow is zero, and there is an airway transmural pressure of 8 cm water.

Finally, at the onset of forced expiration (D), both intrapleural pressure and alveolar pressure increase by 38 cm water (same lung volume as C). Because of the pressure drop along the airway as flow begins, there is now a pressure of 11 cm water, tending to *close* the airway. Airway compression occurs, and the downstream pressure limiting flow becomes the pressure outside the airway, or intrapleural pressure. Thus, the effective driving pressure becomes alveolar minus intrapleural pressure. This is the same Starling resistor mechanism that limits the blood flow in zone 2 of the lung, where venous pressure becomes unimportant just as mouth pressure does here (Figures 4-8 and 4-9). Note that if intrapleural pressure is raised further by increased muscular effort in an attempt to expel gas, the effective driving pressure is unaltered. Thus, flow is independent of effort.

Maximal flow decreases with lung volume (Figure 7-16) because the difference between alveolar and intrapleural pressure decreases and the airways become narrower. Note also that flow is independent of the resistance of the airways downstream of the point of collapse, called the *equal pressure point*. As expiration progresses, the equal pressure point moves distally, deeper into the lung. This occurs because the resistance of the airways rises as lung volume falls,

---

Dynamic Compression of Airways

- Limits air flow in normal subjects during a forced expiration
- May occur in diseased lungs at relatively low expiratory flow rates thus reducing exercise ability
- During dynamic compression flow is determined by alveolar pressure minus pleural pressure (not mouth pressure)
- Is exaggerated in some lung diseases by reduced lung elastic recoil and loss of radial traction on airways

---

and therefore the pressure within the airways falls more rapidly with distance from the alveoli.

Several factors exaggerate this flow-limiting mechanism. One is any increase in resistance of the peripheral airways because that magnifies the pressure drop along them and thus decreases the intrabronchial pressure during expiration (19 cm water in *D*). Another is a low lung volume because that reduces the driving pressure (alveolar-intrapleural). This driving pressure is also reduced if recoil pressure is reduced, as in emphysema. Also in this disease, radial traction on the airways is reduced and they are compressed more readily. Indeed, while this type of flow limitation is only seen during forced expiration in normal subjects, it may occur during the expirations of normal breathing in patients with severe lung disease.

In the pulmonary function laboratory, the flow rate during a maximal expiration is often determined from the *forced expiratory volume* or $FEV_{1.0}$ which is the volume of gas that can be exhaled in 1 second after a maximal inspiration. Another popular measurement is the *forced expiratory flow* or $FEF_{25-75\%}$ which is the average flow rate measured over the middle half (by volume) of the expiration. More information about these tests can be found in Chapter 10.

Causes of Uneven Ventilation

The cause of the regional differences in ventilation in the lung was discussed on p. 103. Apart from these topographical differences, there is some additional inequality of ventilation at any given vertical level in the normal lung, and this is exaggerated in many diseases.

One mechanism of uneven ventilation is shown in Figure 7-19. If we regard a lung unit (Figure 2-1) as an elastic chamber connected to the atmosphere by a tube, the amount of ventilation depends on the compliance of the chamber and the resistance of the tube. In Figure 7-19, unit A has a normal distensibility and airway resistance. It can be seen that its volume change on inspiration is large and rapid so that it is complete before expiration for the whole lung begins (*broken line*). By contrast, unit B has a low compliance, and its change in volume is rapid but small. Finally, unit C has a large airway resistance so that inspiration is slow and not complete before the lung has begun to exhale. Note that the shorter the time available for inspiration (fast breathing rate), the smaller the inspired volume. Such a unit is said to have a long *time constant*, the

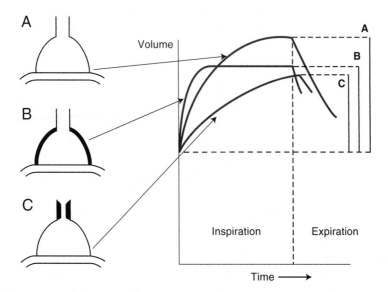

Figure 7-19. Effects of decreased compliance (B) and increased airway resistance (C) on ventilation of lung units compared with normal (A). In both instances, the inspired volume is abnormally low.

value of which is given by the product of the compliance and resistance. Thus, inequality of ventilation can result from alterations in either local distensibility or airway resistance, and the pattern of inequality will depend on the frequency of breathing.

Another possible mechanism of uneven ventilation is incomplete diffusion within the airways of the respiratory zone (Figure 1-4). We saw in Chapter 1 that the dominant mechanism of ventilation of the lung beyond the terminal bronchioles is diffusion. Normally this occurs so rapidly that differences in gas concentration in the acinus are virtually abolished within a fraction of a second. However, if there is dilation of the airways in the region of the respiratory bronchioles, as in some diseases, the distance to be covered by diffusion may be enormously increased. In these circumstances, inspired gas is not distributed uniformly within the respiratory zone because of uneven ventilation *along* the lung units.

Tissue Resistance

When the lung and chest wall are moved, some pressure is required to overcome the viscous forces within the tissues as they slide over each other. Thus, part of the hatched portion of Figure 7-13 should be attributed to these tissue forces. However, this tissue resistance is only about 20% of the total (tissue + airway) resistance in young normal subjects, although it may increase in some diseases. This total resistance is sometimes called *pulmonary resistance* to distinguish it from airway resistance.

Work of Breathing

Work is required to move the lung and chest wall. In this context, it is most convenient to measure work as pressure × volume.

Work Done on the Lung

This can be illustrated on a pressure-volume curve (Figure 7-20). During inspiration, the intrapleural pressure follows the curve ABC, and the work done on the lung is given by the area 0ABCD0. Of this, the trapezoid 0AECD0 represents the work required to overcome the elastic forces, and the hatched area ABCEA represents the work overcoming viscous (airway and tissue) resistance (compare Figure 7-13). The higher the airway resistance or the inspiratory flow rate, the more negative (rightward) would be the intrapleural pressure excursion between A and C and the larger the area.

On expiration, the area AECFA is work required to overcome airway (+ tissue) resistance. Normally, this falls within the trapezoid 0AECD0, and thus this work can be accomplished by the energy stored in the expanded elastic structures and released during a passive expiration. The difference between the areas AECFA and 0AECD0 represents the work dissipated as heat.

The higher the breathing rate, the faster the flow rates and the larger the viscous work area ABCEA. On the other hand, the larger the tidal volume, the larger the elastic work area 0AECD0. It is of interest that patients who have a reduced compliance (stiff lungs) tend to take small rapid breaths, while patients with severe airway obstruction sometimes breathe slowly. These patterns tend to reduce the work done on the lungs.

Figure 7-20. Pressure-volume curve of the lung showing the inspiratory work done overcoming elastic forces (*area 0AECD0*) and viscous forces (*hatched area ABCEA*).

Total Work of Breathing

The total work done moving the lung and chest wall is difficult to measure, although estimates have been obtained by artificially ventilating paralyzed patients (or "completely relaxed" volunteers) in an iron lung type of ventilator. Alternatively, the total work can be calculated by measuring the O_2 cost of breathing and assuming a figure for the efficiency as given by

$$\text{Efficiency \%} = \frac{\text{Useful work}}{\text{Total energy expended (or } O_2 \text{ cost)}} \times 100$$

The efficiency is believed to be about 5 to 10%.

The O_2 cost of quiet breathing is extremely small, being less than 5% of the total resting O_2 consumption. With voluntary hyperventilation it is possible to increase this to 30%. In patients with obstructive lung disease, the O_2 cost of breathing may limit their exercise ability.

QUESTIONS

For each question, choose the one best answer.

1. All of the following statements are true about contraction of the diaphragm **EXCEPT**:
   A. The nerves that are responsible originate high in the neck.
   B. It flattens the diaphragm.
   C. It reduces the lateral distance between the lower rib margins.
   D. It causes the anterior abdominal wall to move out.
   E. It increases lung volume.

2. Which of the following statements about the pressure-volume behavior of the lung is **FALSE**?
   A. Compliance increases with age.
   B. Filling an animal lung with saline increases compliance.
   C. Removing a lobe reduces total pulmonary compliance.
   D. Absence of surfactant reduces compliance.
   E. In the upright lung at FRC, for a given change in intrapleural pressure, the alveoli near the base of the lung expand less than those near the apex.

3. Two bubbles have the same surface tension but bubble X has 3 times the diameter of bubble Y. The ratio of the pressure in bubble X to that in bubble Y is:
   A. 0.3 : 1
   B. 0.9 : 1
   C. 1 : 1
   D. 3 : 1
   E. 9 : 1

4. Pulmonary surfactant is produced by:
   A. Alveolar macrophages.
   B. Goblet cells.
   C. Leukocytes.
   D. Type I alveolar cells.
   E. Type II alveolar cells.

5. The basal regions of the upright human lung are normally better ventilated than the upper regions because:
  A. Airway resistance to the upper regions is higher than to the lower regions.
  B. There is less surfactant in the upper regions.
  C. The blood flow to the lower regions is higher.
  D. The lower regions have a small resting volume and a relatively large increase in volume.
  E. The P_{CO_2} of the lower regions is relatively high.

6. Which of the following statements is **FALSE**? Pulmonary surfactant:
  A. Reduces the surface tension of the alveolar lining liquid.
  B. Is secreted by type II alveolar epithelial cells.
  C. Contains dipalmitoyl phosphatidylcholine.
  D. Increases the work required to expand the lung.
  E. Helps to prevent transudation of fluid from the capillaries into the alveolar spaces.

7. All of the following statements about normal expiration during resting conditions are true **EXCEPT**:
  A. Expiration is generated by the elastic forces.
  B. Alveolar pressure is greater than atmospheric pressure.
  C. Intrapleural pressure gradually falls (becomes more negative) during the expiration.
  D. Flow velocity of the gas (in cm · sec^{-1}) in the large airways exceeds that in the terminal bronchioles.
  E. Diaphragm moves headward as expiration proceeds.

8. An anesthetized patient with paralyzed respiratory muscles and normal lungs is ventilated by positive pressure. If the anesthesiologist increases the lung volume 2 liters above FRC and holds the lung at that volume for 5 seconds, the most likely combination of pressures (in cmH_2O) is likely to be:

	Mouth	Alveolar	Intrapleural
A.	0	0	−5
B.	0	+10	−5
C.	+10	+10	−10
D.	+10	+10	0
E.	+10	0	−10

9. When a normal subject develops a spontaneous pneumothorax of his right lung all of the following occur **EXCEPT**:
  A. Right lung collapses.
  B. Chest wall on the right becomes smaller.
  C. Diaphragm moves down.
  D. Mediastinum may move to the left.
  E. Blood flow to the right lung is reduced.

10. According to Poiseuille's Law reducing the radius of an airway to 1/3 will increase its resistance how many fold?
  A. 1/3
  B. 3
  C. 9

D. 27
E. 81

11. Concerning airflow in the lung:
  A. Flow is more likely to be turbulent in small airways than in the trachea.
  B. The lower the viscosity, the less likely is turbulence to occur.
  C. In pure laminar flow, halving the radius of the airway increases its resistance 8-fold.
  D. For inspiration to occur, mouth pressure must be less than alveolar pressure.
  E. Airway resistance increases during SCUBA diving.

12. The most important factor limiting flow rate during most of a forced expiration from total lung capacity is:
  A. Rate of contraction of expiratory muscles.
  B. Action of diaphragm.
  C. Constriction of bronchial smooth muscle.
  D. Elasticity of chest wall.
  E. Compression of airways.

13. All of the following factors increase the resistance of the airways **EXCEPT**:
  A. Reducing lung volume below FRC.
  B. Increased sympathetic stimulation of airway smooth muscle.
  C. Diving to a great depth.
  D. Inhaling cigarette smoke.
  E. Breathing a mixture of 21% O_2 and 79% sulfur hexafluoride (molecular weight 146).

14. A normal subject makes an inspiratory effort against a closed airway. All of the following statements are true **EXCEPT**:
  A. Tension in the diaphragm increases.
  B. The external intercostal muscles become active.
  C. Intrapleural pressure falls.
  D. Alveolar pressure falls more than intrapleural pressure.
  E. Pressure inside the pulmonary capillaries falls.

8

Control of Ventilation
How Gas Exchange Is Regulated

We have seen that the chief function of the lung is to exchange O_2 and CO_2 between blood and gas and thus maintain normal levels of Po_2 and Pco_2 in the arterial blood. In this chapter we shall see that in spite of widely differing demands for O_2 uptake and CO_2 output made by the body, the arterial Po_2 and Pco_2 are normally kept within close limits. This remarkable regulation of gas exchange is made possible because the level of ventilation is so carefully controlled. First we look at the central controller, and then the various chemoreceptors and other receptors that provide it with information. The integrated responses to carbon dioxide, hypoxia and pH are then described.

121

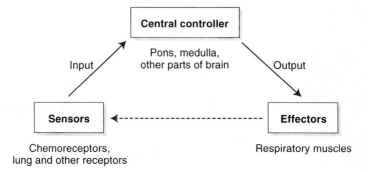

Figure 8-1. Basic elements of the respiratory control system. Information from various sensors is fed to the central controller, the output of which goes to the respiratory muscles. By changing ventilation, the respiratory muscles reduce perturbations of the sensors (negative feedback).

The three basic elements of the respiratory control system (Figure 8-1) are:

1. *Sensors* which gather information and feed it to the
2. *Central controller* in the brain which coordinates the information and, in turn, sends impulses to the
3. *Effectors* (respiratory muscles) which cause ventilation.

We shall see that increased activity of the effectors generally ultimately decreases the sensory input to the brain, for example, by decreasing the arterial P_{CO_2}. This is an example of negative feedback.

Central Controller

The normal automatic process of breathing originates in impulses that come from the brainstem. The cortex can override these centers if voluntary control is desired. Additional input from other parts of the brain occurs under certain conditions.

Brainstem

The periodic nature of inspiration and expiration is controlled by neurons located in the pons and medulla. These have been designated *respiratory centers*. However, these should not be thought of as discrete nuclei but rather as somewhat poorly defined collections of neurons with various components.

Three main groups of neurons are recognized.

1. *Medullary respiratory center* in the reticular formation of the medulla beneath the floor of the fourth ventricle. This comprises two identifiable areas. One group of cells in the dorsal region of the medulla (dorsal respiratory group) is chiefly associated with inspiration; the other in the ventral area (ventral respiratory group) is mainly for expiration. One popular (though not universally ac-

cepted) view is that the cells of the *inspiratory area* have the property of intrinsic periodic firing, and they are responsible for the basic rhythm of ventilation. When all known afferent stimuli have been abolished, these inspiratory cells generate repetitive bursts of action potentials that result in nervous impulses going to the diaphragm and other inspiratory muscles.

The intrinsic rhythm pattern of the inspiratory area starts with a latent period of several seconds during which there is no activity. Action potentials then begin to appear, increasing in a crescendo over the next few seconds. During this time, inspiratory muscle activity becomes stronger in a "ramp"-type pattern. Finally, the inspiratory action potentials cease, and inspiratory muscle tone falls to its preinspiratory level.

The inspiratory ramp can be "turned off" prematurely by inhibiting impulses from the *pneumotaxic center* (see below). In this way, inspiration is shortened and, as a consequence, the breathing rate increases. The output of the inspiratory cells is further modulated by impulses from the vagal and glossopharyngeal nerves. Indeed, these terminate in the tractus solitarius, which is situated close to the inspiratory area.

The *expiratory area* is quiescent during normal quiet breathing because ventilation is then achieved by active contraction of inspiratory muscles (chiefly the diaphragm), followed by passive relaxation of the chest wall to its equilibrium position (Chapter 7). However, in more forceful breathing, for example, on exercise, expiration becomes active as a result of the activity of the expiratory cells. Note that there is still not universal agreement on how the intrinsic rhythmicity of respiration is brought about by the medullary centers.

2. *Apneustic center* in the lower pons. This area is so named because if the brain of an experimental animal is sectioned just above this site, prolonged inspiratory gasps (apneuses) interrupted by transient expiratory efforts are seen. Apparently, the impulses from the center have an excitatory effect on the inspiratory area of the medulla, tending to prolong the ramp action potentials. Whether this apneustic center plays a role in normal human respiration is not known, although in some types of severe brain injury, this type of abnormal breathing is seen.

3. *Pneumotaxic center* in the upper pons. As indicated above, this area appears to "switch off" or inhibit inspiration and thus regulate inspiration volume and, secondarily, respiratory rate. This has been demonstrated experimentally in animals by direct electrical stimulation of the pneumotaxic center. Some investigators believe that the role of this center is "fine tuning" of respiratory rhythm because a normal rhythm can exist in the absence of this center.

Cortex

Breathing is under voluntary control to a considerable extent, and the cortex can override the function of the brainstem within limits. It is not difficult to halve the arterial P_{CO_2} by hyperventilation, although the consequent alkalosis may cause tetany with contraction of the muscles of the hand and foot (carpopedal spasm). Halving the P_{CO_2} increases the arterial pH by about 0.2 unit (Figure 6-8).

Voluntary hypoventilation is more difficult. The duration of breath-holding is limited by several factors, including the arterial P_{CO_2} and P_{O_2}. A preliminary

---

Respiratory Centers

- Responsible for generating the rhythmic pattern of inspiration and expiration
- Located in the medulla and pons of the brain stem
- Receive input from chemoreceptors, lung and other receptors, and the cortex
- Major output is to the phrenic nerves

---

period of hyperventilation increases breath-holding time, especially if oxygen is breathed. However, factors other than chemical are involved. This is shown by the observation that if at the breaking point of breath-holding, a gas mixture is inhaled that *raises* the arterial P_{CO_2} and *lowers* the P_{O_2}, a further period of breath-holding is possible.

Other Parts of the Brain

Other parts of the brain, such as the limbic system and hypothalamus, can alter the pattern of breathing, for example, in emotional states such as rage and fear.

Effectors

The muscles of respiration include the diaphragm, intercostal muscles, abdominal muscles, and accessory muscles such as the sternomastoids. The actions of these were described at the beginning of Chapter 7. In the context of the control of ventilation, it is crucially important that these various muscle groups work in a coordinated manner, and this is the responsibility of the central controller. There is evidence that some newborn children, particularly those that are premature, have uncoordinated respiratory muscle activity, especially during sleep. For example, the thoracic muscles may try to inspire while the abdominal muscles expire. This may be a factor in the "sudden infant death syndrome."

Sensors

Central Chemoreceptors

A chemoreceptor is a receptor that responds to a change in the chemical composition of the blood or other fluid around it. The most important receptors involved in the minute-by-minute control of ventilation are those situated near the ventral surface of the medulla in the vicinity of the exit of the 9th and 10th nerves. In animals, local application of H^+ or dissolved CO_2 to this area stimulates breathing within a few seconds. At one time, it was thought that the medullary respiratory center itself was the site of action of CO_2, but it is now accepted that the chemoreceptors are anatomically separate. Some evidence suggests that they lie about 200 to 400 μm below the ventral surface of the medulla (Figure 8-2).

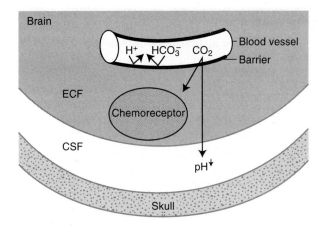

Figure 8-2. Environment of the central chemoreceptors. They are bathed in brain extracellular fluid (ECF), through which CO_2 easily diffuses from blood vessels to cerebrospinal fluid (CSF). The CO_2 reduces the CSF pH, thus stimulating the chemoreceptor. H^+ and HCO_3^- ions cannot easily cross the blood-brain barrier.

The central chemoreceptors are surrounded by brain extracellular fluid and respond to changes in its H^+ concentration. An increase in H^+ concentration stimulates ventilation, whereas a decrease inhibits it. The composition of the extracellular fluid around the receptors is governed by the cerebrospinal fluid (CSF), local blood flow, and local metabolism.

Of these, the CSF is apparently the most important. It is separated from the blood by the blood-brain barrier, which is relatively impermeable to H^+ and HCO_3^- ions, although molecular CO_2 diffuses across it easily. When the blood P_{CO_2} rises, CO_2 diffuses into the CSF from the cerebral blood vessels, liberating H^+ ions which stimulate the chemoreceptors. Thus, the CO_2 level in blood regulates ventilation chiefly by its effect on the pH of the CSF. The resulting hyperventilation reduces the P_{CO_2} in the blood and therefore in the CSF. The cerebral vasodilation that accompanies an increased arterial P_{CO_2} enhances diffusion of CO_2 into the CSF and the brain extracellular fluid.

The normal pH of the CSF is 7.32, and because the CSF contains much less protein than blood, it has a much lower buffering capacity. As a result, the change in CSF pH for a given change in P_{CO_2} is greater than in blood. If the CSF pH is displaced over a prolonged period, a compensatory change in HCO_3^- occurs as a result of transport across the blood-brain barrier. However, the CSF pH does not usually return all the way to 7.32. The change in CSF pH occurs more promptly than the change of the pH of arterial blood by renal compensation (Figure 6-8), a process that takes 2 to 3 days. Because CSF pH returns to near its normal value more rapidly than does blood pH, CSF pH has a more important effect on changes in the level of ventilation and the arterial P_{CO_2}.

One example of these changes is a patient with chronic lung disease and CO_2 retention of long standing who may have a nearly normal CSF pH and, therefore,

---

Central Chemoreceptors

- Located near the ventral surface of the medulla
- Sensitive to the P_{CO_2} but not P_{O_2} of blood
- Respond to the change in pH of the ECF/CSF when CO_2 diffuses out of cerebral capillaries

---

an abnormally low ventilation for his or her arterial P_{CO_2}. A similar situation is seen in normal subjects who are exposed to an atmosphere containing 3% CO_2 for some days.

Peripheral Chemoreceptors

These are located in the carotid bodies at the bifurcation of the common carotid arteries, and in the aortic bodies above and below the aortic arch. The carotid bodies are the most important in humans. They contain glomus cells of two types. Type I cells show an intense fluorescent staining because of their large content of dopamine. These cells are in close apposition to endings of the afferent carotid sinus nerve (Figure 8-3). The carotid body also contains type II cells and a rich supply of capillaries. The precise mechanism of the carotid bodies is still uncertain, but many physiologists believe that the glomus cells are the sites of chemoreception and that modulation of neurotransmitter release from the glomus cells by physiological and chemical stimuli affects the discharge rate of the carotid body afferent fibers (Figure 8-3A).

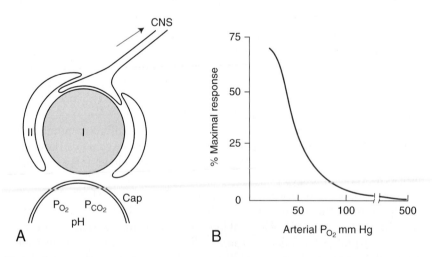

Figure 8-3. A. Diagram of a carotid body which contains type I and type II cells with many capillaries (Cap). Impulses travel to the central nervous system (CNS) through the carotid sinus nerve. **B** shows the nonlinear response to arterial P_{O_2}. Note that the maximum response occurs below a P_{O_2} of 50 mm Hg.

The peripheral chemoreceptors respond to decreases in arterial P_{O_2} and pH, and increases in arterial P_{CO_2}. They are unique among tissues of the body in that their sensitivity to changes in arterial P_{O_2} begins around 500 mm Hg. Figure 8-3B shows that the relationship between firing rate and arterial P_{O_2} is very nonlinear; relatively little response occurs until the arterial P_{O_2} is reduced below 100 mm Hg, but then the rate rapidly increases. The carotid bodies have a very high blood flow for their size, and therefore in spite of their high metabolic rate, the arterial-venous O_2 difference is small. As a result, they respond to arterial rather than to venous P_{O_2}. The response of these receptors can be very fast; indeed, their discharge rate can alter during the respiratory cycle as a result of the small cyclic changes in blood gases. The peripheral chemoreceptors are responsible for all the increase of ventilation that occurs in humans in response to arterial hypoxemia. Indeed, in the absence of these receptors, severe hypoxemia depresses ventilation, presumably through a direct effect on the respiratory centers. Complete loss of hypoxic ventilatory drive has been shown in patients with bilateral carotid body resection.

The response of the peripheral chemoreceptors to arterial P_{CO_2} is less important than that of the central chemoreceptors. For example, when a normal subject is given a CO_2 mixture to breathe, less than 20% of the ventilatory response can be attributed to the peripheral chemoreceptors. However, their response is more rapid, and they may be useful in matching ventilation to abrupt changes in P_{CO_2}.

In humans, the carotid but not the aortic bodies respond to a fall in arterial pH. This occurs regardless of whether the cause is respiratory or metabolic. Interaction of the various stimuli occurs. Thus, increases in chemoreceptor activity in response to decreases in arterial P_{O_2} are potentiated by increases in P_{CO_2} and, in the carotid bodies, by decreases in pH.

Lung Receptors

1. Pulmonary Stretch Receptors

These are also known as slowly adapting pulmonary stretch receptors and are believed to lie within airway smooth muscle. They discharge in response to distension of the lung, and their activity is sustained with lung inflation, that is, they show little adaptation. The impulses travel in the vagus nerve via large myelinated fibers.

The main reflex effect of stimulating these receptors is a slowing of respiratory frequency due to an increase in expiratory time. This is known as the Hering-Breuer inflation reflex. It can be well demonstrated in a rabbit preparation in

---

Peripheral Chemoreceptors

- Located in the carotid and aortic bodies
- Respond to decreased arterial P_{O_2}, increased P_{CO_2} and H^+
- Rapidly responding

which the diaphragm has a slip of muscle from which recordings can be made without interfering with the other respiratory muscles. Classical experiments showed that inflation of the lungs tended to inhibit further inspiratory muscle activity. The opposite response is also seen, that is, deflation of the lungs tends to initiate inspiratory activity (deflation reflex). Thus, these reflexes can provide a self-regulatory mechanism or negative feedback.

The Hering-Breuer reflexes were once thought to play a major role in ventilation by determining the rate and depth of breathing. This could be done by using the information from these stretch receptors to modulate the "switching off" mechanism in the medulla. For example, bilateral vagotomy, which removes the input of these receptors, causes slow, deep breathing in most animals. However, more recent work indicates that the reflexes are largely inactive in adult humans unless the tidal volume exceeds 1 liter, as in exercise. Transient bilateral blockade of the vagi by local anesthesia in awake humans does not change either breathing rate or volume. There is some evidence that these reflexes may be more important in newborn babies.

2. Irritant Receptors

These are thought to lie between airway epithelial cells, and they are stimulated by noxious gases, cigarette smoke, inhaled dusts, and cold air. The impulses travel up the vagus in myelinated fibers, and the reflex effects include bronchoconstriction and hyperpnea. Some physiologists prefer to call these receptors "rapidly adapting pulmonary stretch receptors" because they show rapid adaptation and are apparently involved in additional mechanoreceptor functions, as well as responding to noxious stimuli on the airway walls. It is possible that irritant receptors play a role in the bronchoconstriction of asthma attacks as a result of their response to released histamine.

3. J Receptors

These are the endings of nonmyelimited C fibers and sometimes go by this name. The term "juxta-capillary," or J, is used because these receptors are believed to be in the alveolar walls close to the capillaries. The evidence for this location is that they respond very quickly to chemicals injected into the pulmonary circulation. The impulses pass up the vagus nerve in slowly conducting nonmyelinated fibers and can result in rapid, shallow breathing, although intense stimulation causes apnea. There is evidence that engorgement of pulmonary capillaries and increases in the interstitial fluid volume of the alveolar wall activate these receptors. They may play a role in the rapid, shallow breathing and dyspnea (sensation of difficulty in breathing) associated with left heart failure and interstitial lung disease.

4. Bronchial C-fibers

These are supplied by the bronchial circulation rather than the pulmonary circulation as is the case for J receptors described above. They respond quickly to chemicals injected into the bronchial circulation. The reflex responses to stimulation include rapid shallow breathing, bronchoconstriction, and mucous secretion.

Other Receptors

1. Nose and Upper Airway Receptors

The nose, nasopharynx, larynx, and trachea contain receptors that respond to mechanical and chemical stimulation. These are an extension of the irritant receptors described above. Various reflex responses have been described, including sneezing, coughing, and bronchoconstriction. Laryngeal spasm may occur if the larynx is irritated mechanically, for example, during insertion of an endotracheal tube with insufficient local anesthesia.

2. Joint and Muscle Receptors

Impulses from moving limbs are believed to be part of the stimulus to ventilation during exercise, especially in the early stages.

3. Gamma System

Many muscles, including the intercostal muscles and diaphragm, contain muscle spindles that sense elongation of the muscle. This information is used to reflexly control the strength of contraction. These receptors may be involved in the sensation of dyspnea that occurs when unusually large respiratory efforts are required to move the lung and chest wall, for example, because of airway obstruction.

4. Arterial Baroreceptors

An increase in arterial blood pressure can cause reflex hypoventilation or apnea through stimulation of the aortic and carotid sinus baroreceptors. Conversely, a decrease in blood pressure may result in hyperventilation. The pathways of these reflexes are largely unknown.

5. Pain and Temperature

Stimulation of many afferent nerves can bring about changes in ventilation. Pain often causes a period of apnea followed by hyperventilation. Heating of the skin may result in hyperventilation.

Integrated Responses

Now that we have looked at the various units that make up the respiratory control system (Figure 8-1), it is useful to consider the overall responses of the system to changes in the arterial CO_2, O_2, and pH and to exercise.

Response to Carbon Dioxide

The most important factor in the control of ventilation under normal conditions is the P_{CO_2} of the arterial blood. The sensitivity of this control is remarkable. In the course of daily activity with periods of rest and exercise, the arterial P_{CO_2} is probably held to within 3 mm Hg. During sleep it may rise a little more.

The ventilatory response to CO_2 is normally measured by having the subject inhale CO_2 mixtures or rebreathe from a bag so that the inspired P_{CO_2} gradually rises. In one technique, the subject rebreathes from a bag that is prefilled with 7%

CO_2 and 93% O_2. As the subject rebreathes, metabolic CO_2 is added to the bag, but the O_2 concentration remains relatively high. In such a procedure the P_{CO_2} of the bag gas increases at the rate of about 4 mm Hg/min.

Figure 8-4 shows the results of experiments in which the inspired mixture was adjusted to yield a constant alveolar P_{O_2}. (In this type of experiment on normal subjects, alveolar end-tidal P_{O_2} and P_{CO_2} are generally taken to reflect the arterial levels.) It can be seen that with a normal P_{O_2} the ventilation increases by about 2–3 liters/min for each 1 mm Hg rise in P_{CO_2}. Lowering the P_{O_2} produces two effects: a higher ventilation for a given P_{CO_2}, and the slope of the line becomes steeper. There is considerable variation between subjects.

Another way of measuring respiratory drive is to record the inspiratory pressure during a brief period of airway occlusion. The subject breathes through a mouthpiece attached to a valve box, and the inspiratory port is provided with a shutter. This is closed during an expiration (the subject being unaware), so that the first part of the next inspiration is against an occluded airway. The shutter is opened after about 0.5 sec. The pressure generated during the first 0.1 sec of attempted inspiration (known as $P_{0.1}$) is taken as a measure of respiratory center

Figure 8-4. Ventilatory response to CO_2. Each curve of total ventilation against alveolar P_{CO_2} is for a different alveolar P_{O_2}. In this study, no difference was found between alveolar P_{O_2} values of 110 mm Hg and 169 mm Hg, though some investigators have found that the slope of the line is slightly less at the higher P_{O_2}.

output. This is largely unaffected by the mechanical properties of the respiratory system, although it is influenced by lung volume. This method can be used to study the respiratory sensitivity to CO_2, hypoxia, and other variables as well.

A reduction in arterial P_{CO_2} is very effective in reducing the stimulus to ventilation. For example, if the reader hyperventilates voluntarily for a few seconds, he or she will find that there is no urge to breathe for a short period. An anesthetized patient will frequently stop breathing for a minute or so if first overventilated by the anesthesiologist.

The ventilatory response to CO_2 is reduced by sleep, increasing age, and genetic, racial, and personality factors. Trained athletes and divers tend to have a low CO_2 sensitivity. Various drugs depress the respiratory center, including morphine and barbiturates. Patients who have taken an overdose of one of these drugs often have marked hypoventilation. The ventilatory response to CO_2 is also reduced if the work of breathing is increased. This can be demonstrated by having normal subjects breathe through a narrow tube. The neural output of the respiratory center is not reduced, but it is not so effective in producing ventilation. The abnormally small ventilatory response to CO_2 and the CO_2 retention in some patients with lung disease can be partly explained by the same mechanism. In such patients, reducing the airway resistance with bronchodilators often increases their ventilatory response. There is also some evidence that the sensitivity of the respiratory center is reduced in these patients.

As we have seen, the main stimulus to increase ventilation when the arterial P_{CO_2} rises comes from the central chemoreceptors, which respond to the increased H^+ concentration of the brain extracellular fluid near the receptors. An additional stimulus comes from the peripheral chemoreceptors, because of both the rise in arterial P_{CO_2} and the fall in pH.

Response to Oxygen

The way in which a reduction of P_{O_2} in arterial blood stimulates ventilation can be studied by having a subject breathe hypoxic gas mixtures. The end-tidal P_{O_2} and P_{CO_2} are used as a measure of the arterial values. Figure 8-5 shows that when the alveolar P_{CO_2} is kept at about 36 mm Hg (by altering the inspired mixture), the alveolar P_{O_2} can be reduced to the vicinity of 50 mm Hg before any appreciable increase in ventilation occurs. Raising the P_{CO_2} increases the ventilation at any P_{O_2} (compare Figure 8-4). Note that when the P_{CO_2} is increased, a reduction in P_{O_2} below 100 mm Hg causes some stimulation of ventilation, unlike the

---

Ventilatory Response to Carbon Dioxide

- Arterial P_{CO_2} is the most important stimulus to ventilation under most conditions and it is normally tightly controlled
- Most of the stimulus comes from the central chemoreceptors but the peripheral chemoreceptors also contribute and their response is faster
- The response is magnified if the arterial P_{O_2} is lowered

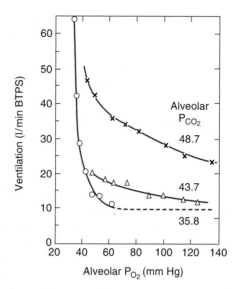

Figure 8-5. Hypoxic response curves. Note that when the P_{CO_2} is 35.8 mm Hg, almost no increase in ventilation occurs until the P_{O_2} is reduced to about 50 mm Hg.

situation in which the P_{CO_2} is normal. Thus, the combined effects of both stimuli exceed the sum of each stimulus given separately, and this is referred to as interaction between the high CO_2 and low O_2 stimuli. Large differences in response occur between individual subjects.

Because the P_{O_2} can normally be reduced so far without evoking a ventilatory response, the role of this hypoxic stimulus in the day-to-day control of ventilation is small. However, on ascent to high altitude, a large increase in ventilation occurs in response to the hypoxia (see Chapter 9).

In some patients with severe lung disease, the hypoxic drive to ventilation becomes very important. These patients have chronic CO_2 retention, and the pH of their brain extracellular fluid has returned to near normal in spite of a raised P_{CO_2}. Thus, they have lost most of their increase in the stimulus to ventilation from CO_2. In addition, the initial depression of blood pH has been nearly abolished by renal compensation so that there is little pH stimulation of the peripheral chemoreceptors (see below). Under these conditions, the arterial hypoxemia becomes the chief stimulus to ventilation. If such a patient is given a high O_2 mixture to breathe to relieve the hypoxemia, ventilation may become grossly depressed. The ventilatory state is best monitored by measuring arterial P_{CO_2}.

As we have seen, hypoxemia reflexly stimulates ventilation by its action on the carotid and aortic body chemoreceptors. It has no action on the central chemoreceptors; indeed, in the absence of peripheral chemoreceptors, hypoxemia depresses respiration. However, prolonged hypoxemia can cause mild cerebral acidosis, which, in turn, can stimulate ventilation.

Ventilatory Response to Hypoxia

- Only the peripheral chemoreceptors are involved
- There is negligible control during normoxic conditions
- The control becomes important at high altitude, and in long-term hypoxemia caused by chronic lung disease

---

Response to pH

A reduction in arterial blood pH stimulates ventilation. In practice, it is often difficult to separate the ventilatory response resulting from a fall in pH from that caused by an accompanying rise in P_{CO_2}. However, in experimental animals in which it is possible to reduce the pH at a constant P_{CO_2}, the stimulus to ventilation can be convincingly demonstrated. Patients with a partly compensated metabolic acidosis (such as uncontrolled diabetes mellitus) who have a low pH and low P_{CO_2} (Figure 6-8) show an increased ventilation. Indeed, this is responsible for the reduced P_{CO_2}.

As we have seen, the chief site of action of a reduced arterial pH is the peripheral chemoreceptors. It is also possible that the central chemoreceptors or the respiratory center itself can be affected by a change in blood pH if it is large enough. In this case, the blood-brain barrier becomes partly permeable to H^+ ions.

Response to Exercise

On exercise, ventilation increases promptly and during strenuous exertion may reach very high levels. Fit young people who attain a maximum O_2 consumption of 4 liters/min may have a total ventilation of 120 liters/min, that is, about 15 times their resting level. This increase in ventilation closely matches the increase in O_2 uptake and CO_2 output. It is remarkable that the cause of the increased ventilation on exercise remains largely unknown.

The arterial P_{CO_2} does not increase during exercise; indeed, during severe exercise it typically falls slightly. The arterial P_{O_2} usually increases slightly, although it may fall at very high work levels. The arterial pH remains nearly constant for moderate exercise, although during heavy exercise it falls because of the liberation of lactic acid through anaerobic glycolysis. It is clear, therefore, that none of the mechanisms we have discussed so far can account for the large increase in ventilation observed during light to moderate exercise.

Other stimuli have been suggested. Passive movement of the limbs stimulates ventilation in both anesthetized animals and awake humans. This is a reflex with receptors presumably located in joints or muscles. It may be responsible for the abrupt increase in ventilation that occurs during the first few seconds of exercise. One hypothesis is that *oscillations in arterial* P_{O_2} *and* P_{CO_2} may stimulate the peripheral chemoreceptors, even though the mean level remains unaltered. These fluctuations are caused by the periodic nature of ventilation and increase when the tidal volume rises, as on exercise. Another theory is that the central chemoreceptors increase ventilation to hold the *arterial* P_{CO_2} constant by some kind of servomechanism, just as the thermostat can control a furnace with little change in temperature. The objection that the arterial P_{CO_2} often *falls* on exercise is countered by the assertion that the preferred level of P_{CO_2} is reset in some way. Proponents of this theory believe that the ventilatory response to inhaled CO_2 may not be a reliable guide to what happens on exercise.

Yet another hypothesis is that ventilation is linked in some way to the additional CO_2 *load* presented to the lungs in the mixed venous blood during exercise. In animal experiments, an increase in this load produced either by infusing CO_2 into the venous blood or by increasing venous return has been shown to correlate well with ventilation. However, a problem with this hypothesis is that no suitable receptor has been found.

Additional factors that have been suggested include the *increase in body temperature* during exercise, which stimulates ventilation, and *impulses from the motor cortex*. However, none of the theories proposed so far is completely satisfactory.

Abnormal Patterns of Breathing

Subjects with severe hypoxemia often exhibit a striking pattern of periodic breathing known as *Cheyne-Stokes respiration*. This is characterized by periods of apnea of 10 to 20 sec, separated by approximately equal periods of hyperventilation when the tidal volume gradually waxes and then wanes. This pattern is frequently seen at high altitude, especially at night during sleep. It is also found in some patients with severe heart disease or brain damage.

The pattern can be reproduced in experimental animals by lengthening the distance through which blood travels on its way to the brain from the lung. Under these conditions, there is a long delay before the central chemoreceptors sense the alteration in P_{CO_2} caused by a change in ventilation. As a result, the respiratory center hunts for the equilibrium condition, always overshooting it. However, not all instances of Cheyne-Stokes respiration can be explained on this basis. Other abnormal patterns of breathing can also occur in disease.

QUESTIONS

For each question, choose the one best answer.

1. Which of the following statements about the respiratory centers is **FALSE**?
   A. The normal rhythmic pattern of breathing originates from neurons in the pons and medulla.
   B. Inspiratory activity originates in the dorsal respiratory group of cells in the medulla.
   C. Impulses from the pneumotaxic center can switch off inspiratory activity.
   D. The cortex of the brain can override the function of the respiratory centers.
   E. The only output from the respiratory centers is via the phrenic nerves.

2. All of the following statements about the central chemoreceptors are true
   EXCEPT:
   A. They are located near the ventral surface of the medulla.
   B. They respond to both the P_{CO_2} and the P_{O_2} of the blood.
   C. They are activated by changes in the pH of the surrounding extracellular
   fluid.
   D. For a given rise in P_{CO_2} the pH of cerebrospinal fluid falls more than that
   of blood.
   E. If the P_{CO_2} of the blood is increased for a long time, the pH of the CSF is
   returned to near normal by movement of bicarbonate into it.

3. Which of the following statements about the peripheral chemoreceptors is
   FALSE?
   A. They respond to changes in arterial P_{O_2}, P_{CO_2} and pH.
   B. Under normoxic conditions the response to changes in P_{O_2} is very small.
   C. The response to changes in P_{CO_2} is faster than for central
   chemoreceptors.
   D. They are the most important receptors causing an increased ventilation
   in response to a rise in P_{CO_2}.
   E. They have a high blood flow per gram of tissue.

4. All of the following statements about the ventilatory response to carbon
   dioxide are true **EXCEPT**:
   A. It is increased if the alveolar P_{O_2} is raised.
   B. It depends on both the peripheral and central chemoreceptors.
   C. It is reduced during sleep.
   D. It is reduced if the work of breathing is increased.
   E. It is a major factor controlling the normal level of ventilation.

5. All of the following statements about the ventilatory response to hypoxia are
   true **EXCEPT**:
   A. It is the major stimulus to ventilation at high altitude.
   B. Ventilation is inhibited if 100% oxygen is breathed.
   C. It increases if the P_{CO_2} is raised.
   D. It may be a major stimulus to ventilation in patients with severe chronic
   lung disease.
   E. It does not play a role in mild carbon monoxide poisoning.

6. The most important stimulus controlling the level of resting ventilation is:
   A. P_{O_2} on peripheral chemoreceptors.
   B. P_{CO_2} on peripheral chemoreceptors.
   C. pH on peripheral chemoreceptors.
   D. pH of CSF on central chemoreceptors.
   E. P_{O_2} on central chemoreceptors.

7. Exercise is one of the most powerful stimulators of ventilation. It primarily
   works by way of:
   A. Low arterial P_{O_2}.
   B. High arterial P_{CO_2}.

    C.   Low P_{O_2} in mixed venous blood.

    D.   Low arterial pH.

    E.   None of the above.

8. All of the following statements about the Hering-Breur inflation reflex are true **EXCEPT**:

    A.   The impulses travel to the brain via the vagus nerve.

    B.   It results in further inspiratory efforts if the lung is maintained inflated.

    C.   It is only seen in adults at high tidal volumes.

    D.   It may help to inflate the newborn lung.

    E.   Abolishing the reflex in many animals causes slow deep breathing.

Respiratory System Under Stress

How Gas Exchange Is Accomplished During Exercise, at Low and High Pressures, and at Birth

The normal lung has enormous reserves at rest, and these enable it to meet the greatly increased demands for gas exchange during exercise. In addition, the lung serves as our principal physiological link with the environment that we live in; its surface area is some 30 times that of the skin. The human urge to climb higher and dive deeper puts the respiratory system under great stress, although these situations are minor insults compared with the process of being born!

Exercise

The gas exchange demands of the lung are enormously increased by exercise. Typically, the resting oxygen consumptions of 300 ml/min can rise to about 3000 ml/min in a moderately fit subject (and as high as 6000 ml/min in an elite athlete). Similarly, the resting CO_2 output of, say, 240 ml/min increases to about 3000 ml/min. Typically, the respiratory exchange ratio (R) rises from about 0.8 at rest to 1.0 on exercise. This increase reflects a greater reliance on carbohydrate rather than fat to produce the required energy. Indeed, R often reaches even higher levels during the unsteady state of severe exercise when lactic acid is produced by anaerobic glycolysis and additional CO_2 is therefore eliminated from bicarbonate. In addition, there is increased CO_2 elimination because the increased H^+ concentration stimulates the peripheral chemoreceptors thus increasing ventilation.

Exercise is conveniently studied on a treadmill or stationary bicycle. As work rate (or power) is increased, oxygen uptake increases linearly (Figure 9-1A). However, above a certain work rate, $\dot{V}_{O_2}$ becomes constant; this is known as the $\dot{V}_{O_2}$max. An increase in work rate above this level can occur only through anaerobic glycolysis.

Ventilation also increases linearly initially when plotted against work rate or $\dot{V}_{O_2}$, but at high $\dot{V}_{O_2}$ values, it increases more rapidly because lactic acid is liberated, and this increases the ventilatory stimulus (Figure 9-1B). Sometimes there is a clear break in the slope, and this has been called *anaerobic threshold,* although the term is somewhat controversial. Unfit subjects produce lactate at relatively low work levels, whereas well-trained subjects can reach fairly high work levels before substantial anaerobic glycolysis occurs.

Many functions of the respiratory system change in response to exercise. The diffusing capacity of the lung increases because of increases in both the diffus-

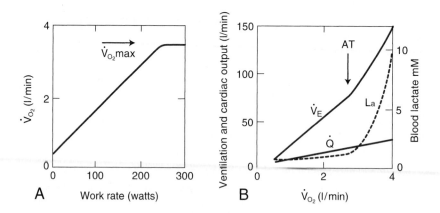

Figure 9-1. A. O_2 consumption ($\dot{V}_{O_2}$) increases nearly linearly with work rate until the $\dot{V}_{O_2}$max is reached. **B.** Ventilation initially increases linearly with O_2 consumption but rises more rapidly when substantial amounts of blood lactate are formed. If there is a clear break, this is sometimes called the anaerobic threshold (AT). Cardiac output increases more slowly than ventilation.

ing capacity of the membrane, D_M, and the volume of blood in the pulmonary capillaries, V_c. These changes are brought about by recruitment and distension of pulmonary capillaries, particularly in the upper parts of the lung. Typically, the diffusing capacity increases at least threefold. Nevertheless, some elite athletes at extremely high work levels show a fall in arterial P_{O_2} caused by diffusion limitation.

Cardiac output increases approximately linearly with work level as a result of increases in both heart rate and stroke volume. However, the change in cardiac output is only about a quarter of the increase in ventilation (in l/min). This makes sense because it is much easier to move air than to move blood. If we look at the Fick equation, $\dot{V}_{O_2} = \dot{Q}(Ca_{O_2} - C\bar{v}_{O_2})$, the increase in $\dot{V}_{O_2}$ is brought about by both an increase in cardiac output and a rise in arterial-venous O_2 difference because of the fall in the oxygen concentration of mixed venous blood. By contrast, if we look at the analogous equation for ventilation, $\dot{V}_{O_2} = \dot{V}_E (F_{I_{O_2}} - F_{E_{O_2}})$, the difference between inspired and expired O_2 concentrations does not change. This is consistent with the much larger increase in ventilation than blood flow. The increase in cardiac output is associated with elevations of both the pulmonary artery and pulmonary venous pressures, which account for the recruitment and distension of pulmonary capillaries. Pulmonary vascular resistance falls.

In normal subjects, the amount of ventilation-perfusion inequality decreases during moderate exercise because of the more uniform topographical distribution of blood flow. However, because the degree of ventilation-perfusion inequality in normal subjects is trivial, this is of little consequence. There is some evidence that in elite athletes at very high work levels, some ventilation-perfusion inequality develops, possibly because of mild degrees of interstitial pulmonary edema. Certainly, fluid must move out of pulmonary capillaries because of the increased pressure within them.

The oxygen dissociation curve moves to the right in exercising muscles because of the increase in P_{CO_2}, H^+ concentration, and temperature. This assists the unloading of oxygen to the muscles. When the blood returns to the lung, the temperature of the blood falls and the curve shifts leftward somewhat. In some animals such as horses and dogs, the hematocrit increases on exercise because red cells are ejected from the spleen, but this does not occur in humans.

In peripheral tissues, additional capillaries open up, thus reducing the diffusion path length to the mitochondria. Peripheral vascular resistance falls because the large increase in cardiac output is not associated with much of an increase in mean arterial pressure, at least during dynamic exercise such as running. During static exercise such as weightlifting, large increases in systemic arterial pressure often occur. Exercise training increases the number of capillaries and mitochondria in skeletal muscle.

As we saw in Chapter 8, the very large increase in ventilation that occurs during exercise is largely unexplained. However, the net result is that the arterial P_{O_2}, P_{CO_2}, and pH are little affected by moderate exercise. At very high work levels, P_{CO_2} often falls, P_{O_2} rises, and pH falls because of lactic acidosis.

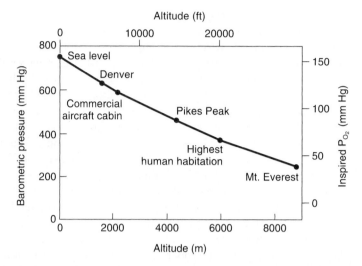

Figure 9-2. Relationship between altitude and barometric pressure. Note that at 1520 m (5000 ft) (Denver, CO), the P_{O_2} of moist inspired gas is about 130 mm Hg, but is only 43 mm Hg on the summit of Mount Everest.

High Altitude

The barometric pressure decreases with distance above the earth's surface in an approximately exponential manner (Figure 9-2). The pressure at 5800 m (19,000 ft) is only one-half the normal 760 mm Hg, so the P_{O_2} of moist inspired gas is $(380 - 47) \times 0.2093 = 70$ mm Hg (47 mm Hg is the partial pressure of water vapor at body temperature). At the summit of Mount Everest (altitude 8848 m or 29,028 ft), the inspired P_{O_2} is only 43 mm Hg. At 19,200 m (63,000 ft), the barometric pressure is 47 mm Hg so that the inspired P_{O_2} is zero.

In spite of the hypoxia associated with high altitude, some 140 million people live at elevations over 2500 m (8000 ft), and permanent residents live higher than 4900 m (16,000 ft) in the Andes. A remarkable degree of acclimatization occurs when humans ascend to these altitudes; indeed, climbers have lived for several days at altitudes that would cause unconsciousness within a few seconds in the absence of acclimatization.

Hyperventilation

The most important feature of acclimatization to high altitude is hyperventilation. Its physiological value can be seen by considering the alveolar gas equation for a climber on the summit of Mount Everest. If the climber's alveolar P_{CO_2} were 40 and respiratory exchange ratio 1, the climber's alveolar P_{O_2} would be $43 - (40/1)^* = 3$ mm Hg! However, by increasing the climber's ventilation five-

---

*When R = 1, the correction factor shown on p. 58 vanishes.

fold, and thus reducing the climber's P_{CO_2} to 8 mm Hg (see p. 18), the climber can raise his or her alveolar P_{O_2} to $43 - 8 = 35$ mm Hg. Typically, the arterial P_{CO_2} in permanent residents at 4600 m (15,000 ft) is about 33 mm Hg.

The mechanism of the hyperventilation is hypoxic stimulation of the peripheral chemoreceptors. The resulting low arterial P_{CO_2} and alkalosis tend to inhibit this increase in ventilation, but after a day or so, the cerebrospinal fluid (CSF) pH is brought partly back by movement of bicarbonate out of the CSF, and after 2 or 3 days, the pH of the arterial blood is returned to near normal by renal excretion of bicarbonate. These brakes on ventilation are then reduced, and it increases further. In addition, there is now evidence that the sensitivity of the carotid bodies to hypoxia increases during acclimatization. Interestingly, people who are born at high altitude have a diminished ventilatory response to hypoxia that is only slowly corrected by subsequent residence at sea level. Conversely, those born at sea level who move to high altitudes retain their hypoxic response intact for a long time. Apparently, therefore, this ventilatory response is determined very early in life.

Polycythemia

Another apparently valuable feature of acclimatization to high altitude is an increase in the red blood cell concentration of the blood. The resulting rise in hemoglobin concentration, and therefore O_2-carrying capacity, means that although the arterial P_{O_2} and O_2 saturation are diminished, the O_2 concentration of the arterial blood may be normal or even above normal. For example, in permanent residents at 4600 m (15,000 ft) in the Peruvian Andes, the arterial P_{O_2} is only 45 mm Hg, and the corresponding arterial O_2 saturation is only 81%. Ordinarily, this would considerably decrease the arterial O_2 concentration, but because of the polycythemia, the hemoglobin concentration is increased from 15 to 19.8 gm/100 ml, giving an arterial O_2 concentration of 22.4 ml/100 ml, which is actually higher than the normal sea level value. The polycythemia also tends to maintain the P_{O_2} of mixed venous blood, and typically in Andean natives living at 4600 m (15,000 ft), this P_{O_2} is only 7 mm Hg below normal (Figure 9-3). The stimulus for the increased production of red blood cells is hypoxemia, which releases erythropoietin from the kidney, which in turn stimulates the bone marrow. Polycythemia is also seen in many patients with chronic hypoxemia caused by lung or heart disease.

Although the polycythemia of high altitude increases the O_2-carrying capacity of the blood, it also raises the blood viscosity. This can be deleterious, and some physiologists believe that the marked polycythemia that is sometimes seen is an inappropriate response.

Other Features of Acclimatization

There is a rightward shift of the O_2 dissociation curve at moderate altitudes that results in a better unloading of O_2 in venous blood at a given P_{O_2}. The cause of the shift is an increase in concentration of 2,3-diphosphoglycerate, which develops primarily because of the respiratory alkalosis. At higher altitudes there is a *leftward shift* in the dissociation curve caused by the respiratory alkalosis, and this assists in the loading of O_2 in the pulmonary capillaries. The *number of capillaries*

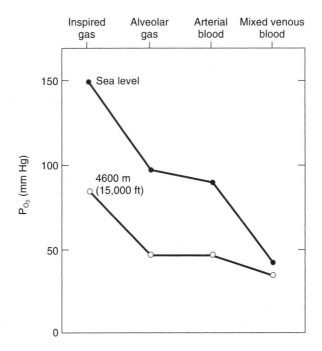

Figure 9-3. P_{O_2} values from inspired air to mixed venous blood at sea level and in residents at an altitude of 4600 m (15,000 ft). Note that in spite of the much lower inspired P_{O_2} at altitude, the P_{O_2} of the mixed venous blood is only 7 mm Hg lower.

per unit volume in peripheral tissues increases, and changes occur in the *oxidative enzymes* inside the cells. The *maximum breathing capacity* increases because the air is less dense, and this assists the very high ventilations (up to 200 liters · min^{-1}) that occur on exercise. However, the maximum O_2 uptake declines rapidly above 4600 m (15,000 ft). This is corrected to a large extent (though not completely) if 100% O_2 is breathed.

Pulmonary vasoconstriction occurs in response to alveolar hypoxia. This increases the pulmonary arterial pressure and the work done by the right heart. The hypertension is exaggerated by the polycythemia which raises the viscosity of the blood. Hypertrophy of the right heart is seen with characteristic changes in the electrocardiogram. There seems to be no physiological advantage in this response, ex-

Acclimatization to High Altitude

- Most important feature is hyperventilation
- Polycythemia is slow to develop and of minor value
- Other features include increases in cellular oxidative enzymes and the concentration of capillaries in some tissues
- Hypoxic pulmonary vasoconstriction is not beneficial

cept that the topographical distribution of blood flow becomes more uniform. The pulmonary hypertension is sometimes associated with pulmonary edema, although the pulmonary venous pressure is normal. The mechanism for this is uncertain, but one hypothesis is that the arteriolar vasoconstriction is uneven, and leakage occurs in unprotected, damaged capillaries. The edema fluid has a high protein concentration, indicating that the permeability of the capillaries is increased.

Newcomers to high altitude frequently complain of headache, fatigue, dizziness, palpitations, insomnia, loss of appetite, and nausea. This is known as *acute mountain sickness* and is attributable to the hypoxemia and alkalosis. Long-term residents sometimes develop an ill-defined syndrome characterized by marked polycythemia, fatigue, reduced exercise tolerance, and severe hypoxemia. This is called *chronic mountain sickness*.

O$_2$ Toxicity

The usual problem is getting enough O$_2$ into the body, but it is possible to have too much. When high concentrations of O$_2$ are breathed for many hours, damage to the lung may occur. If guinea pigs are placed in 100% O$_2$ at atmospheric pressure for 48 hours, they develop pulmonary edema. The first pathological changes are seen in the endothelial cells of the pulmonary capillaries (see Figure 1-1). It is (perhaps fortunately) difficult to administer very high concentrations of O$_2$ to patients, but evidence of impaired gas exchange has been demonstrated after 30 hours of inhalation of 100% O$_2$. Normal volunteers who breathe 100% O$_2$ at atmospheric pressure for 24 hours complain of substernal distress that is aggravated by deep breathing, and they develop a diminution of vital capacity of 500 to 800 ml. This is probably caused by absorption atelectasis (see below).

Another hazard of breathing 100% O$_2$ is seen in premature infants who develop blindness because of retrolental fibroplasia, that is, fibrous tissue formation behind the lens. Here the mechanism is local vasoconstriction caused by the high P$_{O_2}$ in the incubator, and it can be avoided if the arterial P$_{O_2}$ is kept below 140 mm Hg.

Absorption Atelectasis

This is another danger of breathing 100% O$_2$. Suppose that an airway is obstructed by mucus (Figure 9-4). The total pressure in the trapped gas is close to 760 mm Hg (it may be a few mm Hg less as it is absorbed because of elastic forces in the lung). But the sum of the partial pressures in the venous blood is far less than 760 mm Hg. This is because the P$_{O_2}$ of the venous blood remains relatively low, even when O$_2$ is breathed. In fact, the rise in O$_2$ *concentration* of arterial and venous blood when O$_2$ is breathed will be the same if cardiac output remains unchanged, but because of the shape of the O$_2$ dissociation curve (see Figure 6-1), the increase in venous P$_{O_2}$ is only about 10 to 15 mm Hg. Thus, because the sum of the partial pressures in the alveolar gas greatly exceeds that in the venous blood, gas diffuses into the blood, and rapid collapse of the alveoli occurs. Reopening such an atelectatic area may be difficult because of surface tension effects in such small units.

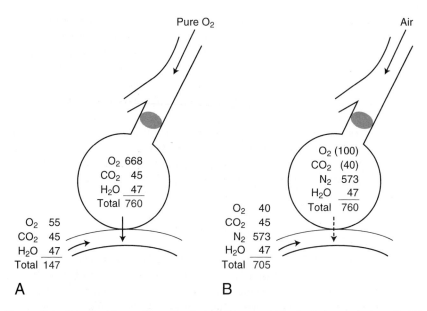

Figure 9-4. Reasons for atelectasis of alveoli beyond blocked airways when O_2 (**A**) and when air (**B**) is breathed. Note that in both cases, the sum of the gas partial pressures in the mixed venous blood is less than in the alveoli. In **B**, the P_{O_2} and P_{CO_2} are shown in *parentheses* because these values change with time. However, the total alveolar pressure remains within a few mm Hg of 760.

Absorption collapse also occurs in a blocked region even when air is breathed, although here the process is slower. Figure 9-4B shows that again the sum of the partial pressures in venous blood is less than 760 mm Hg because the fall in P_{O_2} from arterial to venous blood is much greater than the rise in P_{CO_2} (this is a reflection of the steeper slope of the CO_2 compared with the O_2 dissociation curve—see Figure 6-7). Because the total gas pressure in the alveoli is near 760 mm Hg, absorption is inevitable. Actually, the changes in the alveolar partial pressures during absorption are somewhat complicated, but it can be shown that the rate of collapse is limited by the rate of absorption of N_2. Because this gas has a low solubility, its presence acts as a "splint" that, as it were, supports the alveoli and delays collapse. Even relatively small concentrations of N_2 in alveolar gas have a useful splinting effect. Nevertheless, postoperative atelectasis is a common problem in patients who are treated with high O_2 mixtures. Collapse is particularly likely to occur at the bottom of the lung, where the parenchyma is least well expanded (see Figure 7-8) or the small airways are actually closed (see Figure 7-9). This same basic mechanism of absorption is responsible for the gradual disappearance of a pneumothorax, or a gas pocket introduced under the skin.

Space Flight

The absence of gravity causes a number of physiological changes, and some of these affect the lung. The distribution of ventilation and blood flow become more uniform, with a small corresponding improvement in gas exchange (see Figures 5-8 and 5-10), though some inequality remains because of nongravitational factors. The deposition of inhaled aerosol is altered because of the absence of sedimentation. In addition, thoracic blood volume initially increases because blood does not pool in the legs and this raises pulmonary capillary blood volume and diffusing capacity. Postural hypotension occurs on return to earth; this is known as *cardiovascular deconditioning*. Decalcification of bone and muscle atrophy may occur, presumably through disuse. There is also a small reduction in red cell mass. Space sickness during the first few days of flight can be a serious operational problem.

Increased Pressure

During diving, the pressure increases by 1 atmosphere for every 10 m (33 ft) of descent. Pressure by itself is relatively innocuous, as long as it is balanced.[†] However, if a gas cavity such as the lung, middle ear, or intracranial sinus fails to communicate with the outside, the pressure difference may cause compression on descent or overexpansion on ascent. For example, it is very important for scuba divers to exhale as they ascend to prevent overinflation and possible rupture of the lungs. The increased density of the gas at depth increases the work of breathing. This may result in CO_2 retention, especially on exercise.

Decompression Sickness

During diving, the high partial pressure of N_2 forces this poorly soluble gas into solution in body tissues. This particularly occurs in fat, which has a relatively high N_2 solubility. However, the blood supply of adipose tissue is meager, and the blood can carry little N_2. In addition, the gas diffuses slowly because of its low solubility. As a result, equilibration of N_2 between the tissues and the environment takes hours.

During ascent, N_2 is slowly removed from the tissues. If decompression is unduly rapid, bubbles of gaseous N_2 form, just as CO_2 is released when a bottle of champagne is opened. Some bubbles can occur without physiological disturbances, but large numbers of bubbles cause pain, especially in the region of joints ("bends"). In severe cases, there may be neurological disturbances such as deafness, impaired vision, and even paralysis caused by bubbles in the central nervous system (CNS) that obstruct blood flow.

The treatment of decompression sickness is by recompression. This reduces the volume of the bubbles and forces them back into solution, and often results in a dramatic reduction of symptoms. Prevention is by careful decompression in a series of regulated steps. There are schedules that are based partly on theory and partly on experience and show how rapidly a diver can come up with little risk of developing bends. A short but very deep dive may require hours of gradual decompression. It is now known that bubble formation during ascent is very common. Therefore, the aim of the decompression schedules is to prevent the bubbles from growing too large.

[†] At pressures of hundreds of atmospheres, chemical reactions are affected. For example, the O_2 dissociation curve is displaced.

The risk of decompression sickness following very deep dives can be reduced if a helium-O_2 mixture is breathed during the dive. Helium is about one-half as soluble as N_2 so that less is dissolved in tissues. In addition, it has one-seventh of the molecular weight of N_2 and therefore diffuses more rapidly through tissue (Figure 3-1). Both these factors reduce the risk of bends. Another advantage of a helium-O_2 mixture for divers is its low density, which reduces the work of breathing. Pure O_2 or enriched O_2 mixtures cannot be used at depth because of the dangers of O_2 toxicity (see below).

Commercial divers who are working at great depths, for example on pipelines, sometimes use *saturation diving*. When they are not in the water, they live in a high pressure chamber on the supply ship for several days, which means that they do not return to normal atmospheric pressure during this time. In this way they avoid decompression sickness. However at the end of the period at high pressure, they may take many hours to decompress safely.

Inert Gas Narcosis

Although we usually think of N_2 as a physiological inert gas, at high partial pressures it affects the CNS. At a depth of about 50 m (160 ft) there is a feeling of euphoria (not unlike that following a martini or two), and divers have been known to offer their mouthpieces to fish! At higher partial pressures, loss of coordination and eventually coma may develop.

The mechanism of action is not understood but may be related to the high fat:water solubility of N_2, which is a general property of anesthetic agents. Other gases, such as helium and hydrogen, can be used at much greater depths without narcotic effects.

O_2 Toxicity

We saw earlier that inhalation of 100% O_2 at 1 atmosphere can damage the lung. Another form of O_2 toxicity is stimulation of the CNS, leading to convulsions, when the P_{O_2} considerably exceeds 760 mm Hg. The convulsions may be preceded by premonitory symptoms such as nausea, ringing in the ears, and twitching of the face.

The likelihood of convulsions depends on the inspired P_{O_2} and the duration of exposure, and it is increased if the subject is exercising. At a P_{O_2} of 4 atmospheres, convulsions frequently occur within 30 minutes. For increasingly deep dives, the O_2 concentration is progressively reduced to avoid toxic effects and may eventually be less than 1% for a normal inspired P_{O_2}! The amateur scuba diver should *never* fill his or her tanks with O_2 because of the danger of a convul-

---

Decompression Sickness

- Caused by the formation of N_2 bubbles during ascent from a deep dive
- May result in pain ("bends") and neurological disturbances
- Can be prevented by a slow, staged ascent
- Treated by recompression in a chamber
- Incidence is reduced by breathing a helium-oxygen mixture

sion underwater. However, pure O_2 is sometimes used by the military for shallow dives because a closed breathing circuit with a CO_2 absorber leaves no telltale bubbles. The biochemical basis for the deleterious effects of a high P_{O_2} on the CNS is not fully understood but is probably the inactivation of certain enzymes, especially dehydrogenases containing sulfhydryl groups.

Hyperbaric O_2 Therapy

Increasing the arterial P_{O_2} to a very high level is useful in some clinical situations. One is severe CO poisoning in which most of the hemoglobin is bound to CO and is therefore unavailable to carry O_2. By raising the inspired P_{O_2} to 3 atmospheres in special chambers, the amount of dissolved O_2 in arterial blood can be increased to about 6 ml/100 ml (see Figure 6-1), and thus the needs of the tissues can be met without functioning hemoglobin. Occasionally, an anemic crisis is managed in this way. Hyperbaric O_2 is also useful for treating gas gangrene because the organism cannot live in a high P_{O_2} environment. A hyperbaric chamber is also useful for treating decompression sickness.

Fire and explosions are serious hazards of a 100% O_2 atmosphere, especially at increased pressure. For this reason, O_2 in a pressure chamber is given by mask, and the chamber itself is filled with air.

Polluted Atmospheres[‡]

Atmospheric pollution is an increasing problem in many countries as the number of motor vehicles and industries increases. The chief pollutants are various oxides of nitrogen and sulfur, ozone, carbon monoxide, various hydrocarbons, and particulate matter. Of these, nitrogen oxides, hydrocarbons, and CO are produced in large quantities by the internal combustion engine, the sulfur oxides mainly come from fossil fuel power stations, and ozone is chiefly formed in the atmosphere by the action of sunlight on nitrogen oxides and hydrocarbons. The concentration of atmospheric pollutants is greatly increased by a temperature inversion which prevents the normal escape of the warm surface air to the upper atmosphere.

Nitrogen oxides cause inflammation of the upper respiratory tract and eye irritation, and they are responsible for the yellow haze of smog. Sulfur oxides and ozone also cause bronchial inflammation, and ozone in high concentrations can produce pulmonary edema. The danger of CO is its propensity to tie up hemoglobin (see p. 80), and cyclic hydrocarbons are potentially carcinogenic. Both these pollutants exist in tobacco smoke, which is inhaled in far higher concentrations than any other atmospheric pollutant. There is evidence that some pollutants act synergistically, that is, their combined actions exceed the sum of their individual actions, but more work is required in this area.

Many pollutants exist as *aerosols*, that is, very small particles that remain suspended in the air. When an aerosol is inhaled, its fate depends on the size of the particles. Large particles are removed by *impaction* in the nose and pharynx. This

[‡] For a more detailed account, see JB West: *Pulmonary Pathophysiology—The Essentials*, ed 6. Baltimore, Lippincott Williams & Wilkins, 2003.

means that the particles are unable to turn the corners rapidly because of their inertia, and they impinge on the wet mucosa and are trapped. Medium-sized particles deposit in small airways and elsewhere because of their weight. This is called *sedimentation* and occurs especially where the flow velocity is suddenly reduced because of the enormous increase in combined airway cross section (Figure 1-5). For this reason, deposition is heavy in the terminal and respiratory bronchioles, and this region of a coal miner's lung shows a large dust concentration. The smallest particles (less than 0.1 micron in diameter) reach the alveoli, where some deposition occurs through *diffusion* to the walls. Many small particles are not deposited at all but are exhaled with the next breath.

Once deposited, most of the particles are removed by various clearance mechanisms. Particles that deposit on bronchial walls are swept up the moving staircase of mucus which is propelled by cilia, and they are either swallowed or expectorated. However, the ciliary action can be paralyzed by inhaled irritants. Particles deposited in the alveoli are chiefly engulfed by macrophages that leave via the blood or lymphatics.

Liquid Breathing

It is possible for mammals to survive for some hours breathing liquid instead of air. This was first shown with mice in saline in which the O_2 concentration was increased by exposure to 100% O_2 at 8 atmospheres pressure. Subsequently, mice, rats, and dogs have survived a period of breathing fluorocarbon exposed to pure O_2 at 1 atmosphere. This liquid has a high solubility for both O_2 and CO_2. The animals successfully returned to air breathing.

Because liquids have a much higher density and viscosity than air, the work of breathing is enormously increased. However, adequate oxygenation of the arterial blood can be obtained if the inspired concentration is raised sufficiently. Interestingly, a serious problem is eliminating CO_2. We saw earlier that diffusion within the airways is chiefly responsible for the gas exchange that occurs between the alveoli and the terminal or respiratory bronchioles, where bulk or convective flow takes over. Because the diffusion rates of gases in liquid are many orders of magnitude slower than in the gas phase, this means that a large partial pressure difference for CO_2 between alveoli and terminal bronchioles must be maintained. Animals breathing liquid, therefore, commonly develop CO_2 retention and acidosis. Note that the diffusion pressure of O_2 can always be raised by increasing the inspired P_{O_2}, but this option is not available to help eliminate CO_2. Liquid breathing has been proposed as a possible way of ventilating infants with the respiratory distress syndrome caused by lack of surfactant. The aim is to tide them over the danger period until the surfactant system matures.

Perinatal Respiration

Placental Gas Exchange

During fetal life, gas exchange takes place through the placenta. Its circulation is in parallel with that of the peripheral tissues of the fetus (Figure 9-5) unlike the situation in the adult in which the pulmonary circulation is in series with the systemic circulation. Maternal blood enters the placenta from the uterine arteries and surges into small spaces called intervillous sinusoids which function like the alveoli in the adult. Fetal blood from the aorta is supplied to capillary loops that protrude into the intervillous spaces. Gas exchange occurs across the blood-blood barrier, approximately 3.5 μm thick.

This arrangement is much less efficient for gas exchange than in the adult lung. Maternal blood apparently swirls around the sinusoids somewhat haphazardly, and there are probably large differences of P_{O_2} within these blood spaces. Contrast this situation with the air-filled alveoli in which rapid gaseous diffusion stirs up the alveolar contents. The result is that the P_{O_2} of the fetal blood leaving the placenta is only about 30 mm Hg (Figure 9-5).

This blood mixes with venous blood draining from the fetal tissues and reaches the right atrium (RA) via the inferior vena cava (IVC). Because of streaming within the right atrium, most of this blood then flows directly into the left atrium

Figure 9-5. Blood circulation in the human fetus. The *numbers* show the approximate P_{O_2} of the blood in mm Hg. See text for details.

(LA) through the open foramen ovale (FO) and thus is distributed via the ascending aorta to the brain and heart. Less well oxygenated blood returning to the right atrium via the superior vena cava (SVC) finds its way to the right ventricle (RV), but only a small portion reaches the lungs. Most is shunted to the aorta (Ao) through the ductus arteriosus (DA). The net result of this complex arrangement is that the best oxygenated blood reaches the brain and heart, and the non-gas-exchanging lungs receive only about 15% of the cardiac output. Note that the arterial P_{O_2} in the descending aorta is only about 22 mm Hg.

To summarize the three most important differences between the fetal and adult circulations:

1. The placenta is in parallel with the circulation to the tissues whereas the lung is in series in the adult.
2. The ductus arteriosus shunts most of the blood from the pulmonary artery to the descending aorta.
3. Streaming within the right atrium means that the oxygenated blood from the placenta is preferentially delivered to the left atrium through the foramen ovale and therefore via the aorta to the brain.

The First Breath

The emergence of a baby into the outside world is perhaps the most cataclysmic event of his or her life. The baby is suddenly bombarded with a variety of external stimuli. In addition, the process of birth interferes with placental gas exchange with resulting hypoxemia and hypercapnia. Finally, the sensitivity of the chemoreceptors apparently increases dramatically at birth, although the mechanism is unknown. As a consequence of all these changes, the baby makes the first gasp.

The fetal lung is not collapsed but is inflated with liquid to about 40% of total lung capacity. This fluid is continuously secreted by alveolar cells during fetal life and has a low pH. Some of it is squeezed out as the infant moves through the birth canal, but the remainder has an important role in the subsequent inflation of the lung. As air enters the lung, large surface tension forces have to be overcome. Because the larger the radius of curvature, the lower the pressures (see Figure 7-4), this preinflation reduces the pressures required. Nevertheless, the intrapleural pressure during the first breath may fall to −40 cm water before any air enters the lung, and peak pressures as low as −100 cm water during the first few breaths have been recorded. These very large transient pressures are partly caused by the high viscosity of the lung liquid compared with air. The fetus makes very small, rapid breathing movements in the uterus over a considerable period before birth.

Expansion of the lung is very uneven at first. However, pulmonary surfactant, which is formed relatively late in fetal life, is available to stabilize open alveoli, and the lung liquid is removed by the lymphatics and capillaries. Within a few moments, the functional residual capacity has almost reached its normal value and an adequate gas exchanging surface has been established. However, it is several days before uniform ventilation is achieved.

Changes at or Shortly After Birth

- Baby makes strong inspiratory efforts and takes its first breath
- Large fall in pulmonary vascular resistance
- Ductus arteriosus closes, as does the foramen ovale
- Lung liquid is removed by lymphatics and capillaries

Circulatory Changes

A dramatic fall in pulmonary vascular resistance follows the first few breaths. In the fetus, the pulmonary arteries are exposed to the full systemic blood pressure via the ductus arteriosus, and their walls are very muscular. As a result, the resistance of the pulmonary circulation is exquisitely sensitive to such vasoconstrictor agents as hypoxemia, acidosis, and serotonin and to such vasodilators as acetylcholine. Several factors account for the fall in pulmonary vascular resistance at birth, including the abrupt rise in alveolar P_{O_2} that abolishes the hypoxic vasoconstriction and the increased volume of the lung that widens the caliber of the extra-alveolar vessels (see Figure 4-2).

With the resulting increase in pulmonary blood flow, left atrial pressure rises and the flap-like foramen ovale quickly closes. A rise in aortic pressure resulting from the loss of the parallel umbilical circulation also increases left atrial pressure. In addition, right atrial pressure falls as the umbilical flow ceases. The ductus arteriosus constricts a few minutes later in response to the direct action of the increased P_{O_2} on its smooth muscle. In addition, this constriction is aided by alterations in the levels of local and circulating prostaglandins. Flow through the ductus arteriosus soon reverses as the resistance of the pulmonary circulation falls.

QUESTIONS

For each question, choose the one best answer.

1. All of the following statements about exercise are true **EXCEPT**:
   A. It can increase the oxygen consumption more than tenfold compared with rest.
   B. The measured respiratory exchange ratio may exceed 1.0.
   C. Ventilation increases much more than cardiac output.
   D. At high levels of exercise blood lactate concentrations may rapidly increase.
   E. The change in ventilation on exercise can be explained by the fall in arterial pH.

2. Features of acclimatization to high altitude include all of the following **EXCEPT**:
   A. Hyperventilation.
   B. Polycythemia.
   C. Rightward shift of the O_2 dissociation curve at extreme altitudes.
   D. Increase in the number of capillaries per unit volume in skeletal muscle.
   E. Changes in oxidative enzymes inside muscle cells.

3. If a small airway in a lung is blocked by mucus, the lung distal to this may become atelectatic. Which of the following statements is **FALSE**?
   A. Atelectasis occurs faster if the person is breathing oxygen rather than air.
   B. The sum of the gas partial pressures in mixed venous blood is less than in arterial blood.
   C. The blood flow to the atelectatic region will fall.
   D. The same mechanism explains the absorption of a spontaneous pneumothorax.
   E. The elastic properties of the lung strongly resist atelectasis.

4. Helium-oxygen mixtures rather than nitrogen-oxygen mixtures (with the same oxygen concentration) are preferable for very deep diving because all of the following are reduced **EXCEPT**:
   A. Risk of decompression sickness.
   B. Work of breathing.
   C. Airway resistance.
   D. Risk of O_2 toxicity.
   E. Risk of inert gas narcosis.

5. The absence of gravity during spaceflight alters all of the following **EXCEPT**:
   A. Distribution of pulmonary blood flow.
   B. Distribution of ventilation.
   C. Deposition of inhaled aerosol particles.
   D. Thoracic blood volume.
   E. Work of breathing.

6. Which of the following increases by the largest percentage at maximal exercise compared with rest?
   A. Heart rate.
   B. Alveolar ventilation.
   C. P_{CO_2} of mixed venous blood.
   D. Cardiac output.
   E. Tidal volume.

7. The transition from placental to pulmonary gas exchange is accompanied by all of the following **EXCEPT**:
   A. Increased arterial P_{O_2}.
   B. Fall of pulmonary vascular resistance.
   C. Closure of the ductus arteriosus.
   D. Reversal of blood flow through the foramen ovale.
   E. Strong respiratory efforts.

Tests of Pulmonary Function
How Respiratory Physiology Is Applied to Measure Lung Function*

This final chapter deals with pulmonary function testing which is an important practical application of respiratory physiology in the clinic. First we look at the forced expiration, a very simple but nevertheless very useful test. Then there are sections on ventilation-perfusion relationships, blood gases, lung mechanics, control of ventilation and the role of exercise. The chapter concludes by emphasizing that it is more important to understand the principles of respiratory physiology contained in Chapters 1–9 than to concentrate on the details of pulmonary function tests.

* This chapter is only a brief introduction to pulmonary function tests. A more detailed description can be found in JB West: *Pulmonary Pathophysiology—The Essentials*, ed 6. Baltimore, Lippincott, Williams & Wilkins, 2003.

An important practical application of respiratory physiology is the testing of pulmonary function. These tests are useful in a variety of settings. The most important is the hospital pulmonary function laboratory or, on a small scale, the physician's office, where these tests help in the diagnosis and the management of patients with pulmonary or cardiac diseases. In addition, they may be valuable in deciding whether a patient is fit enough for surgery. Another use is the evaluation of disability for the purposes of insurance and worker's compensation. Again, some of the simpler tests are employed in epidemiological surveys to assess industrial hazards or to document the prevalence of disease in the community.

The role of pulmonary function tests should be kept in perspective. They are rarely a key factor in making a definitive diagnosis in a patient with lung disease. Rather, the various patterns of impaired function overlap disease entities. While the tests are often valuable for following the progress of a patient with chronic pulmonary disease and assessing the results of treatment, it is generally far more important for the medical student (or physician) to understand the principles of how the lung works (Chapters 1 through 9) than to concentrate only on lung function tests.

Ventilation

Forced Expiration

A very useful and simple test of pulmonary function is the measurement of a single forced expiration. Figure 10-1 shows the spirometer record obtained when a subject inspires maximally and then exhales as hard and as completely as he or she can. The volume exhaled in the first second is called the forced expiratory volume, or $FEV_{1.0}$, and the total volume exhaled is the forced vital capacity, or FVC (this is often slightly less than the vital capacity measured on a slow exhalation as in Figure 2-2). Normally, the $FEV_{1.0}$ is about 80% of the FVC.

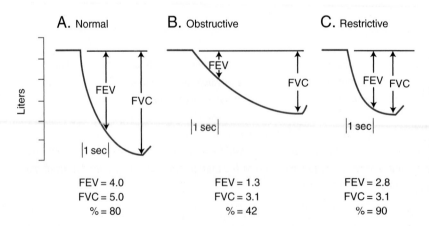

Figure 10-1. Measurement of forced expiratory volume ($FEV_{1.0}$) and forced vital capacity (FVC).

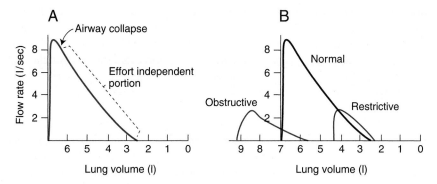

Figure 10-2. Flow volume curve obtained by recording flow rate against volume during a forced expiration from maximum inspiration. The figure shows absolute lung volumes, although these cannot be measured from single expirations.

In disease, two general patterns can be distinguished. In *restrictive* diseases such as pulmonary fibrosis, both FEV and FVC are reduced, but characteristically the $FEV_{1.0}/FVC\%$ is normal or increased. In *obstructive* diseases such as bronchial asthma, the $FEV_{1.0}$ is reduced much more than the FVC, giving a low FEV/FVC%. Frequently, mixed restrictive and obstructive patterns are seen.

A related measurement is the *forced expiratory flow rate*, or $FEF_{25-75\%}$, which is the average flow rate measured over the middle half of the expiration. Generally, this is closely related to the $FEV_{1.0}$, although occasionally it is reduced when the $FEV_{1.0}$ is normal. Sometimes other indices are also measured from the forced expiration curve.

A useful way of looking at forced expirations is with *flow-volume curves* (see Figure 7-16). Figure 10-2 reminds us that after a relatively small amount of gas has been exhaled, flow is limited by airway compression and is determined by the elastic recoil force of the lung and the resistance of the airways upstream of the collapse point. In *restrictive diseases*, the maximum flow rate is reduced, as is the total volume exhaled. However, if flow is related to the absolute lung volume (that is, including the residual volume which cannot be measured from a single expiration), the flow rate is often abnormally high during the latter part of expiration because of the increased lung recoil (Figure 10-2B). By contrast, in *obstructive* diseases the flow rate is very low in relation to lung volume, and a scooped-out appearance is often seen following the point of maximum flow.

What is the significance of these measurements of forced expirations? The FVC may be reduced at its top or bottom end (see Figure 10-2). In *restrictive*

Forced Expiration Test

- Measures the FEV and the FVC
- Simple to do and often informative
- Distinguishes between obstructive and restrictive disease

diseases, inspiration is limited by the reduced compliance of the lung or chest wall, or weakness of the inspiration muscles. In *obstructive* disease, the total lung capacity is typically abnormally large, but expiration ends prematurely. The reason for this is early airway closure brought about by increased smooth muscle tone of the bronchi, as in asthma, or loss of radial traction from surrounding parenchyma, as in emphysema. Other causes include edema of the bronchial walls, or secretions within the airways.

The $FEV_{1.0}$ (or $FEF_{25-75\%}$) is reduced by an increase in airway resistance or a reduction in elastic recoil of the lung. It is remarkably independent of expiratory effort. The reason for this is the dynamic compression of airways, which was discussed earlier (see Figure 7-18). This mechanism explains why the flow rate is independent of the resistance of the airways downstream of the collapse point but is determined by the elastic recoil pressure of the lung and the resistance of the airways upstream of the collapse point. The location of the collapse point is in the large airways, at least initially. Thus, both the increase in airway resistance and the reduction of lung elastic recoil pressure can be important factors in the reduction of the $FEV_{1.0}$, as, for example, in pulmonary emphysema.

Lung Volumes

The determination of lung volumes by spirometry and the measurement of functional residual capacity (FRC) by helium dilution and body plethysmography were discussed earlier (see Figures 2-2 through 2-4). The FRC can also be found by having the subject breathe 100% O_2 for several minutes and washing all the N_2 out of the subject's lung.

Suppose that the lung volume is V_1 and that the total volume of gas exhaled over 7 minutes is V_2 and that its concentration of N_2 is C_2. We know that the concentration of N_2 in the lung before washout was 80%, and we can measure the concentration left in the lung by sampling end-expired gas with an N_2 meter at the lips. Call this concentration C_3. Then, assuming no net change in the amount of N_2, we can write $V_1 \times 80 = (V_1 \times C_3) + (V_2 \times C_2)$. Thus, V_1 can be derived. A disadvantage of this method is that the concentration of nitrogen in the gas collected over 7 minutes is very low, and a small error in its measurement leads to a larger error in calculated lung volume. In addition, some of the N_2 that is washed out comes from body tissues, and this should be allowed for. This method, like the helium dilution technique, measures only ventilated lung volume, whereas, as we saw on p. 16, the body plethysmograph method includes gas trapped behind closed airways.

The measurement of anatomic dead space by Fowler's method was described earlier (see Figure 2-6).

Diffusion

The principles of the measurement of the diffusing capacity for carbon monoxide by the single breath method were discussed on p. 31. The diffusing capacity for O_2 is very difficult to measure, and it is only done as a research procedure.

Blood Flow

The measurement of total pulmonary blood flow by the Fick principle and by the indicator dilution method was alluded to on p. 42.

Ventilation-Perfusion Relationships

Topographical Distribution of Ventilation and Perfusion

Regional differences of ventilation and blood flow can be measured using radioactive xenon, as briefly described earlier (see Figures 2-7 and 4-7).

Inequality of Ventilation

This can be measured by single breath and multiple breath methods. The *single breath method* is very similar to that described by Fowler for measuring anatomic dead space (Figure 2-6). There we saw that if the N_2 concentration at the lips is measured following a single breath of O_2, the N_2 concentration of the expired alveolar gas is almost uniform, giving a nearly flat "alveolar plateau." This reflects the approximately uniform dilution of the alveolar gas by the inspired O_2. By contrast, in patients with lung disease, the alveolar N_2 concentration continues to rise during expiration. This is caused by the uneven dilution of the alveolar N_2 by inspired O_2.

The reason why the concentration rises is that the poorly ventilated alveoli (those in which the N_2 has been diluted least) always empty last, presumably because they have long time constants (Figures 7-19 and 10-5). In practice, the change in N_2 percentage concentration between 750 and 1250 ml of expired volume is often used as an index of uneven ventilation. This is a simple, quick, and useful test.

The *multiple breath* method is based on the rate of washout of N_2 as shown in Figure 10-3. The subject is connected to a source of 100% O_2, and a fast-responding N_2 meter samples gas at the lips. If the ventilation of the lung were uniform, the N_2 concentration would be reduced by the same *fraction* with each breath. For example, if the tidal volume (excluding dead space) were equal to the FRC, the N_2 concentration would halve with each breath. In general, the N_2 concentration is $FRC/[FRC + (V_T - V_D)]$ times that of the previous breath, where V_T and V_D are the tidal volume and anatomic dead space, respectively. Because the N_2 is reduced by the same fraction with each breath, the plot of log N_2 concentration against breath number would be a straight line (see Figure 10-3) if the lung behaved as a single, uniformly ventilated compartment. This is very nearly the case in normal subjects.

In patients with lung disease, however, the nonuniform ventilation results in a curved plot because different lung units have their N_2 diluted at different rates. Thus, fast ventilated alveoli cause a rapid initial fall in N_2, whereas slow ventilated spaces are responsible for the long tail of the washout (see Figure 10-3).

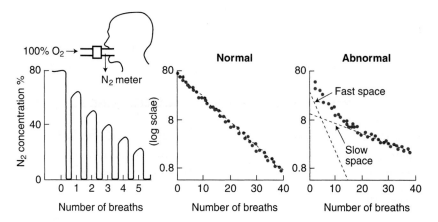

Figure 10-3. N$_2$ washout obtained when a subject breathes 100% O$_2$. Normal lungs give an almost linear plot of N$_2$ concentration against number of breaths on semilogarithmic paper, but this plot is nonlinear when uneven ventilation is present.

Inequality of Ventilation-Perfusion Ratios

One way of assessing the mismatch of ventilation and blood flow within the diseased lung is that introduced by Riley. This is based on measurements of P$_{O_2}$ and P$_{CO_2}$ in arterial blood and expired gas (the principles were briefly described in Chapter 5). In practice, expired gas and arterial blood are collected simultaneously from the patient, and various indices of ventilation-perfusion inequality are computed.

One useful measurement is the *alveolar-arterial P$_{O_2}$ difference*. We saw in Figure 5-11 how this develops because of regional differences of gas exchange in the normal lung. Figure 10-4 is an O$_2$-CO$_2$ diagram that allows us to examine this development more closely. First, suppose that there is no ventilation-perfusion inequality and that all the lung units are represented by a single point (i) on the ventilation-perfusion line. This is known as the "ideal" point. Now as ventilation-perfusion inequality develops, the lung units begin to spread away from i toward both v̄ (low ventilation-perfusion ratios) and I (high ventilation-perfusion ratios) (compare Figure 5-7). When this happens, the mixed capillary blood (a) and mixed alveolar gas (A) also diverge from i. They do so along lines i to v̄ and i to I, which represent a constant respiratory exchange ratio (CO$_2$ output/O$_2$ uptake), as this is determined by the metabolism of the body tissues.[†]

The horizontal distance between A and a represents the *(mixed) alveolar-arterial O$_2$ difference*. In practice, this can only be measured easily if ventilation is essentially uniform but blood flow is uneven, because only then can a represen-

---

[†] In this necessarily simplified description, some details are omitted. For example, the mixed venous point alters when ventilation-perfusion inequality develops.

Figure 10-4. O_2-CO_2 diagram showing the ideal point (i), that is, the hypothetical composition of alveolar gas and end-capillary blood when no ventilation-perfusion inequality is present. As inequality develops, the arterial (a) and alveolar (A) points diverge along their respective R (respiratory exchange ratio) lines. The mixed alveolar-arterial P_{O_2} difference is the horizontal distance between the points.

tative sample of mixed alveolar gas be obtained. This is sometimes the case in pulmonary embolism. More frequently, the P_{O_2} difference between ideal alveolar gas and arterial blood is calculated—the (*ideal*) *alveolar-arterial O_2 difference*. The ideal alveolar P_{O_2} can be calculated from the alveolar gas equation which relates the P_{O_2} of any lung unit to the composition of the inspired gas, the respiratory exchange ratio, and the P_{CO_2} of the unit. In the case of ideal alveoli, the P_{CO_2} is taken to be the same as arterial blood because the line along which point i moves is so nearly horizontal. Note that this alveolar-arterial P_{O_2} difference is caused by units between i and $\bar{v}$, that is, those with low ventilation-perfusion ratios.

Two more indices of ventilation-perfusion inequality are frequently derived. One is *physiologic shunt* (also called *venous admixture*). For this we pretend that all of the leftward movement of the arterial point (a) away from the ideal point (i) (that is, the hypoxemia) is caused by the addition of mixed venous blood ($\bar{v}$) to ideal blood (i). This is not so fanciful as it first seems, because units with very low ventilation-perfusion ratios put out blood that has essentially the same composition as mixed venous blood (see Figures 5-6 and 5-7). In practice, the shunt equation (see Figure 5-3) is used in the following form:

$$\frac{\dot{Q}_{PS}}{\dot{Q}_T} = \frac{Ci_{O_2} - Ca_{O_2}}{Ci_{O_2} - C\bar{v}_{O_2}}$$

where $\dot{Q}_{PS}/\dot{Q}_T$ refers to the ratio of the physiologic shunt to total flow. The O_2 concentration of ideal blood is calculated from the ideal P_{O_2} and O_2 dissociation curve.

The other index is *alveolar dead space*. Here we pretend that all of the movement of the alveolar point (A) away from the ideal point (i) is caused by the addition of inspired gas (I) to ideal gas. Again, this is not such an outrageous notion as it may first appear because units with very high ventilation-perfusion ratios behave very much like point I. After all, a unit with an infinitely high ventilation-perfusion ratio contains gas that has the same composition as inspired air (see Figures 5.6 and 5.7). The Bohr equation for dead space (see p. 19) is used in the following form:

$$\frac{V_{D_{alv}}}{V_T} = \frac{P_{I_{CO_2}} - P_{A_{CO_2}}}{P_{I_{CO_2}}}$$

where A refers to expired alveolar gas. The result is called *alveolar dead space* to distinguish it from the *anatomic dead space*, that is, the volume of the conducting airways. Because expired alveolar gas is often difficult to collect without contamination by the anatomic dead space, the mixed expired CO_2 is often measured. The result is called the *physiologic dead space*, which includes components from the alveolar dead space and anatomic dead space. Because the P_{CO_2} of ideal gas is very close to that of arterial blood (see Figure 10-4), the equation for physiologic dead space is

$$\frac{V_{D_{phys}}}{V_T} = \frac{P_{a_{CO_2}} - P_{E_{CO_2}}}{P_{a_{CO_2}}}$$

The normal value for physiologic dead space is about 30% of the tidal volume at rest and less on exercise, and it consists almost completely of anatomic dead space. In lung disease it may increase to 50% or more due to the presence of ventilation-perfusion inequality.

Blood Gases and pH

P_{O_2}, P_{CO_2}, and pH are easily measured in blood samples with blood gas electrodes. A glass electrode is used to measure the pH of whole blood. The P_{CO_2} electrode is, in effect, a tiny pH meter in which a bicarbonate buffer solution is separated from the blood sample by a thin membrane. When carbon dioxide diffuses across the membrane from the blood, the pH of the buffer changes in accordance with the Henderson-Hasselbalch relationship. The pH meter then reads out the P_{CO_2}. The O_2 electrode is a polarograph, that is, a device which, when supplied with a suitable voltage, gives a minute current that is proportional to the amount of dissolved O_2. In practice, all three electrodes are arranged to give their outputs on the same meter by appropriate switching, and a complete analysis on a blood sample can be done in a few minutes.

We saw in Chapter 5 that there are four causes of low arterial P_{O_2} or hypoxemia: (1) hypoventilation, (2) diffusion impairment, (3) shunt, and (4) ventilation-perfusion inequality.

In distinguishing between these causes keep in mind that hypoventilation is *always* associated with a raised arterial P_{CO_2} and that only when a shunt is present does the arterial P_{O_2} fail to rise to the expected level when 100% O_2 is administered. In diseased lungs, impaired diffusion is always accompanied by ventilation-perfusion inequality, and, indeed, it is usually impossible to determine how much of the hypoxemia is attributable to defective diffusion.

There are two causes of an increased arterial P_{CO_2}: (1) hypoventilation, and (2) ventilation-perfusion inequality. The latter does not *always* cause CO_2 retention because any tendency for the arterial P_{CO_2} to rise signals the respiratory center via the chemoreceptors to increase ventilation and thus hold the P_{CO_2} down. However, in the absence of this increased ventilation, the P_{CO_2} must rise. Changes in the blood gases in different types of hypoxemia are summarized in Table 6.1.

The assessment of the acid-base status of the blood was discussed on pp. 86–87.

Mechanics of Breathing

Lung Compliance

Compliance is defined as the volume change per unit of pressure change across the lung. To obtain this, we need to know intrapleural pressure. In practice, esophageal pressure is measured by having the subject swallow a small balloon on the end of a catheter. Esophageal pressure is not identical to intrapleural pressure but reflects its pressure changes fairly well. The measurement is not reliable in supine subjects because of interference by the weight of the mediastinal structures.

A simple way of measuring compliance is to have the subject breathe out from total lung capacity into a spirometer in steps of, say, 500 ml and measure his or her esophageal pressure simultaneously. The glottis should be open, and the lung should be allowed to stabilize for a few seconds after each step. In this way, a pressure-volume curve similar to the upper line in Figure 7-3 is obtained. The whole curve is the most informative way of reporting the elastic behavior of the lung. Indices of the shape of the curve can be derived. Notice that the compliance, which is the slope of the curve, will vary depending on what lung volume is used. It is conventional to report the slope over the liter above FRC measured during deflation. Even so, the measurement is not very repeatable.

Lung compliance can also be measured during resting breathing, as shown in Figure 7-13. Here we make use of the fact that at no-flow points (end of inspiration or expiration), the intrapleural pressure reflects only the elastic recoil forces and not those associated with airflow. Thus, the volume difference divided by the pressure difference at these points is the compliance.

This method is not valid in patients with airway disease because the variation in time constants throughout the lung means that flow still exists within the lung when it has ceased at the mouth. Figure 10-5 shows that if we consider a lung region that has a partially obstructed airway, it will always lag behind the rest of the lung (compare Figure 7-19). In fact, it may continue to fill when the rest of the lung has begun to empty, with the result that gas moves into it from adjoining lung units—so called *pendelluft* (swinging air). As the breathing frequency is increased, the proportion of the tidal volume that goes to this partially obstructed region becomes smaller and smaller. Thus, less and less of the

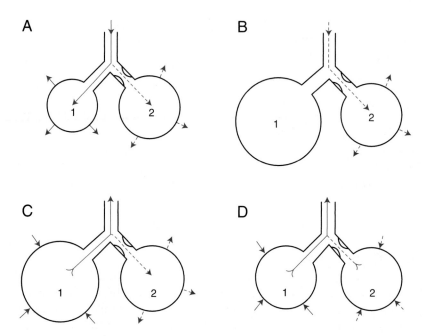

Figure 10-5. Effects of uneven time constants on ventilation. Compartment 2 has a partially obstructed airway and, therefore, a long time constant (compare Figure 7-19). During inspiration (**A**), gas is slow to enter it, and it therefore continues to fill after the rest of the lung (1) has stopped moving (**B**). Indeed at the beginning of the expiration (**C**), the abnormal region (2) may still be inhaling while the rest of the lung has begun to exhale. In **D**, both regions are exhaling but compartment 2 lags behind compartment 1. At higher frequencies, the tidal volume to the abnormal region becomes progressively smaller.

lung is participating in the tidal volume changes, and therefore the lung appears to become less compliant.

Airway Resistance

This is the pressure difference between the alveoli and the mouth per unit of airflow (Figure 7-12). It can be measured in a body plethysmograph (Figure 10-6).

Before inspiration (A), the box pressure is atmospheric. At the onset of inspiration, the pressure in the alveoli falls as the alveolar gas expands by a volume ΔV. This compresses the gas in the box and from its change in pressure ΔV can be calculated (compare Figure 2-4). If lung volume is known, ΔV can be converted into alveolar pressure using Boyle's law. Flow is measured simultaneously, and thus airway resistance is obtained. The measurement is made during expiration in the same way. Lung volume is determined as described in Figure 2-4.

Airway resistance can also be measured during normal breathing from an intrapleural pressure record as obtained with an esophageal balloon (see Figure 7-13). However, in this case, tissue viscous resistance is included as well (see p. 116). Intrapleural pressure reflects two sets of forces, those opposing the elastic recoil of the lung and those overcoming resistance to air and tissue flow. It is possible to subtract the pressure caused by the recoil forces during quiet breathing because this is proportional to lung volume (if compliance is constant). The subtraction is done with an electrical circuit. We are then left with a plot of pressure against flow which gives (airway + tissue) resistance. This method is not satisfactory in lungs with severe airway disease because the uneven time constants prevent all regions from moving together (see Figure 10-5).

Closing Volume

Early disease in small airways can be sought by using the single breath N_2 washout (see Figure 2-6) and thus exploiting the topographical differences of ventilation (see Figures 7-8 and 7-9). Suppose a subject takes a vital capacity breath of 100% O_2 and during the subsequent exhalation the N_2 concentration at the lips is measured (Figure 10-7). Four phases can be recognized.

First, pure dead space is exhaled (1) followed by a mixture of dead space and alveolar gas (2), and then pure alveolar gas (3). Toward the end of expiration, an abrupt increase in N_2 concentration is seen (4). This signals closure of airways at the base of the lung (see Figure 7-9), and is caused by preferential emptying of the apex, which has a relatively high concentration of N_2. The reason for the higher N_2 at the apex is that during a vital capacity breath of O_2, this region expands less (see Figure 7-9), and, therefore, the N_2 there is less diluted with O_2. Thus, the volume of the lung at which dependent airways begin to close can be read off the tracing.

In young normal subjects, the closing volume is about 10% of the vital capacity (VC). It increases steadily with age and is equal to about 40% of the VC, that is the FRC, at about the age of 65 years. Relatively small amounts of disease in the small airways apparently increase the closing volume. Sometimes the *closing capacity* is reported. This is the closing volume plus the residual volume.

Figure 10-6. Measurement of airway resistance with the body plethysmograph. During inspiration, the alveolar gas is expanded, and box pressure therefore rises. From this, alveolar pressure can be calculated. The difference between alveolar and mouth pressure, divided by flow, gives airway resistance (see text).

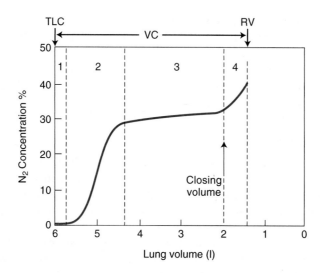

Figure 10-7. Measurement of the closing volume. If a vital capacity inspiration of 100% O_2 is followed by a full expiration, four phases in the N_2 concentration measured at the lips can be recognized (see text). The last is caused by preferential emptying of the apex of the lung after the lower zone airways have closed.

Control of Ventilation

The responsiveness of the chemoreceptors and respiratory center to CO_2 can be measured by having the subject rebreathe into a rubber bag, as discussed on p. 129. We saw that the alveolar P_{O_2} also affects ventilation so that if the response to CO_2 alone is required, the inspired P_{O_2} should be kept above 200 mm Hg to avoid any hypoxic drive. The ventilatory response to hypoxia can be measured in a similar way if the subject rebreathes from a bag with a low P_{O_2} but constant P_{CO_2}.

Exercise

Additional information about pulmonary function can often be obtained if tests are made when the subject exercises. As discussed at the beginning of Chapter 9, the resting lung has enormous reserves; its ventilation, blood flow, O_2 and CO_2 transfer, and diffusing capacity can be increased severalfold on exercise. Frequently, patients with early disease have pulmonary function tests that are within normal limits at rest, but abnormalities are revealed when the respiratory system is stressed by exercise.

Methods of providing controlled exercise include the treadmill and bicycle ergometer. Measurements most often made on exercise include total ventilation, pulse rate, O_2 uptake, CO_2 output, respiratory exchange ratio, arterial blood gases, and the diffusing capacity of the lung for carbon monoxide.

Perspective on Tests of Pulmonary Function

In this chapter, we have touched on some of the lung function tests that are presently available. In conclusion, it should be emphasized that not all these tests are commonly used in a hospital pulmonary function laboratory. Only a few can be used in a doctor's office or on an epidemiological survey.

The most useful and simple test in the clinical setting is the *forced expiration*. It does not matter much which indices are derived from this test, but the $FEV_{1.0}$ and FVC are very frequently reported. Next, the ability to measure *arterial blood gases* is essential if patients with respiratory failure are managed and is valuable in any case. After these, the relative importance of tests becomes more a matter of personal preference, but a well-equipped pulmonary function laboratory would be able to measure lung volumes, inequality of ventilation, alveolar-arterial P_{O_2} difference, physiologic dead space and shunt, diffusing capacity for carbon monoxide, airway resistance, lung compliance, ventilatory response to CO_2 and hypoxia, and the patient's response to exercise. In large laboratories, more specialized measurements such as the topographical distribution of ventilation and blood flow would be available.

QUESTIONS

For each question, choose the one best answer.

1. Which of the following statements about the 1 second forced expiratory volume is **FALSE**?
   A. It can be used to assess the efficacy of bronchodilators.
   B. It is reduced by dynamic compression of the airways.
   C. It is reduced in patients with chronic obstructive pulmonary disease but not pulmonary fibrosis.
   D. It is reduced in patients with asthma.
   E. The test is easy to perform.

2. All of the following may reduce the FEV_1 in a patient with chronic obstructive pulmonary disease **EXCEPT**:
   A. Hypertrophy of the diaphragm.
   B. Excessive secretions in the airways.
   C. Reduction in the number of small airways.
   D. Loss of radial traction on the airways.
   E. Loss of elastic recoil of the lung.

3. All of the following statements are true of the single breath nitrogen test for uneven ventilation **EXCEPT**:
   A. The slope of the alveolar plateau is increased in chronic bronchitis.
   B. The slope occurs because poorly ventilated units empty later in expiration than well-ventilated units.
   C. The last exhaled gas comes from the apex of the lung.
   D. A similar procedure can be used to measure the anatomic dead space.
   E. The test is very time consuming.

4. In the assessment of ventilation-perfusion inequality based on measurements of P_{O_2} and P_{CO_2} in arterial blood and expired gas, all of the following statements are true **EXCEPT**:

  A. The ideal alveolar P_{O_2} is calculated using the arterial P_{CO_2}.

  B. The alveolar P_{O_2} is then calculated from the alveolar gas equation.

  C. $\dot{V}_A/\dot{Q}$ inequality increases the alveolar-arterial P_{O_2} difference.

  D. $\dot{V}_A/\dot{Q}$ inequality increases the physiologic shunt.

  E. $\dot{V}_A/\dot{Q}$ inequality reduces the physiologic dead space.

5. A seated normal subject exhales to residual volume (RV).

  A. The volume of gas remaining in the lung is more than half of the vital capacity.

  B. The P_{CO_2} of the expired gas falls just before the end of expiration.

  C. If the mouthpiece is closed at RV and the subject completely relaxes, the pressure in the airways is greater than atmospheric pressure.

  D. Intrapleural pressure exceeds alveolar pressure at RV.

  E. All small airways in the lung are closed at RV.

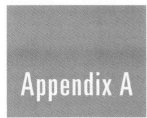

Appendix A

Symbols, Units, and Equations

Symbols

Primary Symbols

C   Concentration of gas in blood
F   Fractional concentration in dry gas
P   Pressure or partial pressure
Q   Volume of blood
$\dot{Q}$ Volume of blood per unit time
R   Respiratory exchange ratio
S   Saturation of hemoglobin with O_2
V   Volume of gas
$\dot{V}$ Volume of gas per unit time

Secondary Symbols for Gas Phase

A   Alveolar
B   Barometric
D   Dead space
E   Expired
I   Inspired
L   Lung
T   Tidal

Secondary Symbols for Blood Phase

a   arterial
c   capillary
c′   end-capillary
i   ideal
v   venous
$\bar{v}$ mixed venous

Examples

O_2 concentration in arterial blood Ca_{O_2}
Fractional concentration of N_2 in expired gas Fe_{N_2}
Partial pressure of O_2 in mixed venous blood $P\bar{v}_{O_2}$

Units

Traditional metric units have been used in this book. Pressures are given in mm Hg; the torr is an almost identical unit.

In Europe, SI (Système International) units are commonly used. Most of these are familiar, but the kilopascal, the unit of pressure, is confusing at first. One kilopascal = 7.5 mm Hg (approximately).

Equations

Gas Laws

General gas law: $PV = RT$

where T is temperature and R is a constant. This equation is used to correct gas volumes for changes of water vapor pressure and temperature. For example, ventilation is conventionally reported at BTPS, that is, body temperature (37°C), ambient pressure, and saturated with water vapor because it then corresponds to the volume changes of the lung. By contrast, gas volumes in blood are expressed as STPD, that is, standard temperature (0°C or 273°K) and pressure (760 mm Hg) and dry, as is usual in chemistry. To convert a gas volume at BTPS to one at STPD, multiply by

$$\frac{273}{310} \times \frac{P_B - 47}{760}$$

where 47 mm Hg is the water vapor pressure at 37°C.

Boyle's law $\qquad\qquad P_1V_1 = P_2V_2$ (temperature constant)

and *Charles' law* $\qquad\qquad \dfrac{V_1}{V_2} = \dfrac{T_1}{T_2}$ (pressure constant)

are special cases of the general gas law.

Avogadro's law states that equal volumes of different gases at the same temperature and pressure contain the same number of molecules. A gram molecule, for example, 32 gm of O_2, occupies 22.4 liters at STPD.

Dalton's law states that the partial pressure of a gas (x) in a gas mixture is the pressure that this gas would exert if it occupied the total volume of the mixture in the absence of the other components.

Thus, $P_x = P \cdot F_x$, where P is the total dry gas pressure, since F_x refers to dry gas. In gas with a water vapor pressure of 47 mm Hg

$$P_x = (P_B - 47) \cdot F_x$$

Also, in the alveoli, $P_{O_2} + P_{CO_2} + P_{N_2} + P_{H_2O} = P_B$.

The *partial pressure of a gas in solution* is its partial pressure in a gas mixture that is in equilibrium with the solution.

Henry's law states that the concentration of gas dissolved in a liquid is proportional to its partial pressure. Thus, $C_x = K \cdot P_x$.

Ventilation

$$V_T = V_D + V_A$$

where V_A here refers to the volume of alveolar gas in the tidal volume

$$\dot{V}_A = \dot{V}_E - \dot{V}_D$$

$$\dot{V}_{CO_2} = \dot{V}_A \cdot F_{ACO_2} \text{ (both } \dot{V} \text{ measured at BTPS)}$$

$$\dot{V}_A = \frac{\dot{V}_{CO_2}}{P_{ACO_2}} \times K \text{ (alveolar ventilation equation)}$$

If $\dot{V}_A$ is BTPS and $\dot{V}_{CO_2}$ is STPD, K = 0.863. In normal subjects, P_{ACO_2} is nearly identical to P_{aCO_2}.

   Bohr equation

$$\frac{V_D}{V_T} = \frac{P_{ACO_2} - P_{ECO_2}}{P_{ACO_2}}$$

Or, using arterial P_{CO_2},

$$\frac{V_D}{V_T} = \frac{P_{aCO_2} - P_{ECO_2}}{P_{aCO_2}}$$

This gives *physiologic dead space*.

Diffusion

In the *gas phase*, *Graham's law* states that the rate of diffusion of a gas is inversely proportional to the square root of its molecular weight.

   In *liquid or a tissue slice*, *Fick's law** states that the volume of gas per unit time which diffuses across a tissue sheet is given by

$$\dot{V}_{gas} = \frac{A}{T} \cdot D \cdot (P_1 - P_2)$$

where A and T are the area and thickness of the sheet, P_1 and P_2 are the partial pressure of the gas on the two sides, and D is a diffusion constant sometimes called the permeability coefficient of the tissue for that gas.

   This *diffusion constant* is related to the solubility (Sol) and the molecular weight (MW) of the gas

$$D \propto \frac{Sol}{\sqrt{MW}}$$

When the diffusing capacity of the lung (D_L) is measured with carbon monoxide and the capillary P_{CO} is taken at zero,

$$D_L = \frac{\dot{V}_{CO}}{P_{ACO}}$$

---

* Fick's law was originally expressed in terms of concentrations, but partial pressures are more convenient for us.

D_L is made up of two components. One is the diffusing capacity of the alveolar membrane (D_M), and the other depends on the volume of capillary blood (V_c) and the rate of reaction of CO with hemoglobin θ

$$\frac{1}{D_L} = \frac{1}{D_M} + \frac{1}{\theta \cdot V_c}$$

Blood Flow

Fick principle

$$\dot{Q} = \frac{\dot{V}_{O_2}}{Ca_{O_2} - C\bar{v}_{O_2}}$$

Pulmonary vascular resistance

$$PVR = \frac{P_{art} - P_{ven}}{\dot{Q}}$$

where P_{art} and P_{ven} are the mean pulmonary arterial and venous pressures, respectively.

Starling's law of fluid exchange across the capillaries

$$\text{Net flow out} = K[(P_c - P_i) - \sigma(\pi_c - \pi_i)]$$

where i refers to the interstitial fluid around the capillary, π refers to the colloid osmotic pressure, σ is the reflection coefficient, and K is the filtration coefficient.

Ventilation-Perfusion Relationships

Alveolar gas equation

$$P_{A_{O_2}} = P_{I_{O_2}} - \frac{P_{A_{CO_2}}}{R} + \left[P_{A_{CO_2}} \cdot F_{I_{O_2}} \cdot \frac{1 - R}{R}\right]$$

This is only valid if there is no CO_2 in inspired gas. The term in square brackets is a relatively small correction factor when air is breathed (2 mm Hg when $P_{CO_2} = 40$, $F_{I_{O_2}} = 0.21$, and R = 0.8). Thus, a useful approximation is

$$P_{A_{O_2}} = P_{I_{O_2}} - \frac{P_{A_{CO_2}}}{R}$$

Respiratory exchange ratio
If no CO_2 is present in the inspired gas

$$R = \frac{\dot{V}_{CO_2}}{\dot{V}_{O_2}} = \frac{P_{E_{CO_2}}(1 - F_{I_{O_2}})}{P_{I_{O_2}} - P_{E_{O_2}} - (P_{E_{CO_2}} \cdot F_{I_{O_2}})}$$

Venous to arterial shunt

$$\frac{\dot{Q}_S}{\dot{Q}_T} = \frac{Cc'_{O_2} - Ca_{O_2}}{Cc'_{O_2} - C\bar{v}_{O_2}}$$

where c' means end-capillary.

Ventilation-perfusion ratio equation

$$\frac{\dot{V}_A}{\dot{Q}} = \frac{8.63\ R(Ca_{O_2} - C\bar{v}_{O_2})}{Pa_{CO_2}}$$

where blood gas concentrations are in $ml \cdot 100\ ml^{-1}$.

Physiologic shunt

$$\frac{\dot{Q}_{PS}}{\dot{Q}_T} = \frac{Ci_{O_2} - Ca_{O_2}}{Ci_{O_2} - C\bar{v}_{O_2}}$$

Alveolar dead space

$$\frac{V_D}{V_T} = \frac{Pi_{CO_2} - Pa_{CO_2}}{Pi_{CO_2}}$$

The equation for *physiologic dead* space is on p. 160.

Blood Gases and pH

O_2 dissolved in blood

$$C_{O_2} = Sol \cdot P_{O_2}$$

where Sol is $0.003\ ml\ O_2 \cdot 100\ ml\ blood^{-1} \cdot mm\ Hg^{-1}$.

Henderson-Hasselbalch equation

$$pH = pK_A + \log \frac{(HCO_3^-)}{(CO_2)}$$

The pK_A for this system is normally 6.1. If HCO_3^- and CO_2 concentrations are in millimoles per liter, CO_2 can be replaced by P_{CO_2} (mm Hg) $\times$ 0.030.

Mechanics of Breathing

Compliance $= \Delta V/\Delta P$

Specific compliance $= \Delta V/(V \cdot \Delta P)$

Laplace equation for pressure caused by surface tension of a sphere

$$P = \frac{2T}{r}$$

where r is the radius. Note that for a soap bubble, $P = 4T/r$, because there are two surfaces.

Poiseuille's law for laminar flow

$$\dot{V} = \frac{P\pi r^4}{8nl}$$

where n is the coefficient of viscosity[†] and P is the pressure difference across the length l.

Reynolds number

$$Re = \frac{2rvd}{n}$$

where v is average linear velocity of the gas, d is its density, and n is its viscosity.

Pressure drop for laminar flow, $P\alpha\dot{V}$, but for turbulent flow, $P\alpha\dot{V}^2$ (approximately).

Airway resistance

$$\frac{P_{alv} - P_{mouth}}{\dot{V}}$$

where P_{alv} and P_{mouth} refer to alveolar and mouth pressures, respectively.

[†] This is a corruption of the Greek letter η for those of us who have little Latin and less Greek.

Appendix B

Answers

Chapter 1

1. E
2. B
3. B
4. D
5. B
6. A

Chapter 2

1. B
2. E
3. C
4. D
5. B
6. B

Chapter 3

1. C
2. E
3. E
4. A
5. A
6. D

Chapter 4

1. D
2. C
3. E
4. E
5. C
6. E
7. D
8. A
9. A
10. E

Chapter 5

1. D
2. B
3. A
4. B
5. B
6. E
7. A
8. E
9. D

Chapter 6

1. D
2. E
3. E
4. E
5. A
6. E
7. B
8. C
9. A
10. A
11. E
12. E

Chapter 7

1. C
2. E
3. A
4. E
5. D
6. D
7. C
8. D
9. B

10. E
11. E
12. E
13. B
14. D

Chapter 8

1. E
2. B
3. D
4. A
5. B
6. D
7. E
8. B

Chapter 9

1. E
2. C
3. E
4. D
5. E
6. B
7. D

Chapter 10

1. C
2. A
3. E
4. E
5. B

Further Reading

Most of the material in this book is very basic and the original papers go back many years. A good place to find more recent work is one of the encyclopedic textbooks such as *The Lung: Scientific Foundations*, ed 2, edited by RG Crystal, JB West, PJ Barnes and ER Weibel, New York, Lippincott-Raven Press, 1997. The following list includes some of the classical papers and books.

Structure and Function

DEJOURS P: *Principles of Comparative Respiratory Physiology*. Amsterdam, North Holland, 1975.
HAYEK H VON: *The Human Lung*, translated by VE Krahl. New York, Hafner, 1960.
MURRAY JF: *The Normal Lung*, ed 2. Philadelphia, WB Saunders, 1986.
WEIBEL ER: *Morphometry of the Human Lung*. New York, Academic Press, 1963.
WEIBEL ER: *The Pathway for Oxygen*. Cambridge, Mass., Harvard University Press, 1984.

Ventilation

CUMMING G, CRANK J, HORSFIELD K, PARKER I: Gaseous diffusion in the airways of the human lung. *Respir Physiol* 1:58–74, 1966.
FOWLER WS: Intrapulmonary distribution of inspired gas. *Physiol Rev* 32:1–20, 1952.
HLASTALA MP: Ventilation. In RG Crystal, JB West, PJ Barnes, ER Weibel (eds): *The Lung: Scientific Foundations*, ed 2. New York, Lippincott-Raven Press, 1997.
PAIVA M: Uneven ventilation. In RG Crystal, JB West, PJ Barnes, ER Weibel (eds): *The Lung: Scientific Foundations*, ed 2. New York, Lippincott-Raven Press, 1997.

Diffusion

FORSTER RE: Diffusion of gases across the alveolar membrane. In Farhi L, Tenney SM (eds): *Handbook of Physiology. The Respiratory System*. Bethesda, MD, American Physiological Society, 1987, vol 4, sect 3, pp 71–88.
KROGH M: The diffusion of gases through the lungs of man. *J Physiol (Lond)* 49:271–300, 1914–1915.
ROUGHTON FJW, FORSTER RE: Relative importance of diffusion and chemical reaction rates in determining rate of exchange of gases in the human lung, with special reference to true diffusing capacity of pulmonary membrane and volume of blood in the lung capillaries. *J Appl Physiology* 11:290–302, 1957.
SCHEID P, PIIPER J: Diffusion. In RG Crystal, JB West, PJ Barnes, ER Weibel (eds): *The Lung: Scientific Foundations*, ed 2. New York, Lippincott-Raven Press, 1997.
WAGNER PD: Diffusion and chemical reaction in pulmonary gas exchange. *Physiol Rev* 57:257–312, 1977.

Blood Flow and Metabolism

FUNG YC, SOBIN SS: Theory of sheet flow in lung alveoli. *J Appl Physiol* 26:472–488, 1969.

GLAZIER JB, HUGHES JMB, MALONEY JE, WEST JB: Measurements of capillary dimensions and blood volume in rapidly frozen lungs. *J Appl Physiol* 26:65–76, 1969.

HUGHES JMB, MORRELL NW: Pulmonary circulation: from basic mechanisms to clinical practice. London, Imperial College Press, 2001.

LEE G, DUBOIS AB: Pulmonary capillary blood flow in man. *J Clin Invest* 34:1380–1390, 1955.

PERMUTT S, RILEY RL: Hemodynamics of collapsible vessels with tone: the vascular waterfall. *J Appl Physiol* 18:924–932, 1963.

SILVERMAN ES, GERRITSEN ME, COLLINS T: Metabolic function of the pulmonary endothelium. In RG Crystal, JB West, PJ Barnes, ER Weibel (eds): *The Lung: Scientific Foundations*, ed 2. New York, Lippincott-Raven Press, 1997.

WEST JB, DOLLERY CT, NAIMARK A: Distribution of blood flow in isolated lung: relation to vascular and alveolar pressures. *J Appl Physiol* 19:713–724, 1964.

Ventilation-Perfusion Relationships

RAHN H, FENN WO: *A Graphical Analysis of the Respiratory Gas Exchange. The O_2-CO_2 Diagram*. Washington, DC, American Physiological Society, 1955.

RILEY RL, COURNAND A: "Ideal" alveolar air and the analysis of ventilation-perfusion relationships in the lungs. *J Appl Physiol* 1:825–847, 1949.

RILEY RL, COURNAND A: Analysis of factors affecting partial pressures of oxygen and carbon dioxide in gas and blood of lungs: theory. *J Appl Physiol* 4:77–101, 1951.

WEST JB: *Ventilation/Blood Flow and Gas Exchange*, ed 5. Oxford, Blackwell, 1990.

WEST JB, WAGNER PD: Ventilation-perfusion relationships. In RG Crystal, JB West, PJ Barnes, ER Weibel (eds): *The Lung: Scientific Foundations*, ed 2. New York, Lippincott-Raven Press, 1997.

Gas Transport by the Blood

BAUMANN R: Blood oxygen transport. In Farhi L, Tenney SM (eds): *Handbook of Physiology. The Respiratory System*. Bethesda, MD, American Physiology Society, 1987, vol 4, sect 3, pp 147–172.

DAVENPORT HW: *The ABC of Acid Base Chemistry*, ed 6. Chicago, University of Chicago Press, 1974.

JONES NL: Acid-base physiology. In RG Crystal, JB West, PJ Barnes, ER Weibel (eds): *The Lung: Scientific Foundations*, ed 2. New York, Lippincott-Raven Press, 1997.

KLOCKE RA: Carbon dioxide transport. In RG Crystal, JB West, PJ Barnes, ER Weibel (eds): *The Lung: Scientific Foundations*, ed 2. New York, Lippincott-Raven Press, 1997.

ROUGHTON FJW: Transport of oxygen and carbon dioxide. In Fenn WO, Rahn H (eds): *Handbook of Physiology. Respiratory*. Washington, DC, American Physiological Society, 1964, vol 1, sect 3, pp 767–826.

SEVERINGHAUS JW: Electrodes for blood and gas P_{CO_2}, P_{O_2} and blood pH. *Acta Anesthesiol Scand* (Suppl.) 11:207–220, 1962.

Mechanics of Breathing

DE TROYER A: The respiratory muscles. In RG Crystal, JB West, PJ Barnes, ER Weibel (eds): *The Lung: Scientific Foundations*, ed 2. New York, Lippincott-Raven Press, 1997.

GOERKE J, SCHURCH S: Mechanical properties of the alveolar surface. In RG Crystal, JB West, PJ Barnes, ER Weibel (eds): *The Lung: Scientific Foundations*, ed 2. New York, Lippincott-Raven Press, 1997.

HOPPIN FG, HILDEBRANDT J: Mechanical properties of the lung. In West JB (ed): *Bioengineering Aspects of the Lung*. New York, Dekker, 1977.

MILIC-EMILI J, HENDERSON JAM, DOLOVICH MB, TROP D, KANEKO K: Regional distribution of inspired gas in the lung. *J Appl Physiol* 21:749–759, 1966.

PEDLEY TJ, SCHROTER RC, SUDLOW MF: Gas flow and mixing in airways. In West JB (ed): *Bioengineering Aspects of the Lung*. New York, Dekker, 1977.

PRIDE NB, PERMUTT S, RILEY RL, BROMBERGER-BARNEA B: Determinants of maximum expiratory flow from the lungs. *J Appl Physiol* 23:646–662, 1967.

RAHN H, OTIS AB, CHADWICK LE, FENN WO: The pressure-volume diagram of the thorax and lung. *Am J Physiol* 146:161–178, 1946.

Control of Ventilation

CHERNIACK NS, WIDDICOMBE JG (eds): Control of breathing. In *Handbook of Physiology. The Respiratory System*. Bethesda, MD, American Physiological Society, 1986, vol 2, sect 3.

CUNNINGHAM DJC, LLOYD BB (eds): *The Regulation of Human Respiration*. Oxford, Blackwell, 1963.

HORNBEIN TF (ed): *Regulation of Breathing*. New York, Dekker, 1981.

HOWELL JBL, CAMPBELL EJM: *Breathlessness*. Philadelphia, Davis, 1966.

PORTER R (ed): *Hering-Breuer Centenary Symposium*. Ciba Foundation Symposium. London, Churchill, 1970.

VON EULER C. Neural organization and rhythm generation. In RG Crystal, JB West, PJ Barnes, ER Weibel (eds): *The Lung: Scientific Foundations*, ed 2. New York, Lippincott-Raven Press, 1997.

Respiratory System Under Stress

BARCROFT J: *The Respiratory Function of the Blood. Part I. Lessons from High Altitude*. London, Cambridge University Press, 1925.

BERT P: *Barometric Pressure. Researches in Experimental Physiology* 1878, translated by MA Hitchcock and FA Hitchcock. Columbus, Ohio, College Book Co., 1943.

DAWES GS: *Foetal and Neonatal Physiology: A Comparative Study of the Changes at Birth*. Chicago, Year Book, 1968.

HURTADO A: Animals in high altitudes: resident man. In Dill DB (ed): *Handbook of Physiology. Adaptation to the Environment*. Washington, DC, American Physiological Society, 1964, sect 4, pp 843–860.

MCARDLE WD, KATCH FI, KATCH VL: *Exercise Physiology*. ed 5. Philadelphia, Lippincott, Williams and Wilkins, 2001.

STOLP BW, LUNDGREN CEG, PIANTADOSI CA: Diving and immersion. In RG Crystal, JB West, PJ Barnes, ER Weibel (eds): *The Lung: Scientific Foundations*, ed 2. New York, Lippincott-Raven Press, 1997.

WARD MP, MILLEDGE JS, WEST JB: *High Altitude Medicine and Physiology*, ed 3. London, Arnold, 2000.

Tests of Pulmonary Function

COTES JE: *Lung Function: Assessment and Application in Medicine*, ed 5. Oxford, Blackwell, 1993.

HUGHES JMB, PRIDE NB: *Lung function tests*. London, Saunders, 1999.

WEST JB: *Pulmonary Pathophysiology—The Essentials*, ed 6. Baltimore, Lippincott, Williams & Wilkins, 2003.

Figure Credits

Figure 1-1   From Weibel ER: *Respir Physiol* 11:54, 1970.

Figure 1-2   Scanning electron micrograph by Nowell JA, Tyler WS.

Figure 1-4   Modified From Weibel ER: *The Pathway for Oxygen*. Cambridge: Harvard University Press, 1984, p. 275.

Figure 1-6   From Maloney JE, Castle BL: *Respir Physiol* 7:150, 1969.

Figure 1-7   From Glazier JB, et al: *J Appl Physiol* 26:65, 1969.

Figure 2-1   Modified from West JB: *Ventilation/Blood Flow and Gas Exchange*, ed 5. Oxford: Blackwell, 1990, p. 3.

Figure 4-2   From Hughes JMB, et al: *Respir Physiol* 4:58, 1968.

Figure 4-7   Redrawn from Hughes JMB, et al: *Respir Physiol* 4:58, 1968.

Figure 4-8   From West JB, et al: *J Appl Physiol* 19:713, 1964.

Figure 4-10   From Barer GR, et al: *J Physiol* 211:139, 1970.

Figure 5-2   Modified from West JB: *Ventilation/Blood Flow and Gas Exchange*, ed 5. Oxford: Blackwell, 1990, p-3.

Figure 5-5   From West JB: *Ventilation/Blood Flow and Gas Exchange*, ed 5. Oxford: Blackwell, 1990.

Figure 5-6   From West JB: *Ventilation/Blood Flow and Gas Exchange*, ed 5. Oxford: Blackwell, 1990.

Figure 5-7   From West JB: *Ventilation/Blood Flow and Gas Exchange*, ed 5. Oxford: Blackwell, 1990.

Figure 5-8   From West JB: *Ventilation/Blood Flow and Gas Exchange*, ed 5. Oxford: Blackwell, 1990.

Figure 5-9   From West JB: *Ventilation/Blood Flow and Gas Exchange*, ed 5. Oxford: Blackwell, 1990.

Figure 5-11   From West JB: *Lancet* 2:1055, 1963.

Figure 5-12   Modified from West JB: *Ventilation/Blood Flow and Gas Exchange*, ed 5. Oxford: Blackwell, 1990.

Figure 5-13   Redrawn from Wagner et al: *J Clin Invest* 54:54, 1974.

Figure 5-14   Redrawn from Wagner et al: *J Clin Invest* 54:54, 1974.

Figure 7-5   From Radford EP: *Tissue Elasticity*. Washington, DC: American Physiological Society, 1957.

Figure 7-6   From Weibel ER, Gil J: In West JB: *Bioengineering Aspects of the Lung*. New York: Marcel Dekker, 1977.

Figure 7-8   From West JB: *Ventilation/Blood Flow and Gas Exchange*, ed. 5. Oxford: Blackwell, 1990.

Figure 7-9   From West JB: *Ventilation/Blood Flow and Gas Exchange*, ed. 5. Oxford: Blackwell, 1990.

Figure 7-14   Redrawn from Pedley TJ, et al: *Respir Physiol* 9:387, 1970.

Figure 7-15   Redrawn from Briscoe WA, Dubois AB: *J Clin Invest* 37:1279, 1958.

Figure 7-17   Redrawn from Fry DL, Hyatt RE: *Am J Med* 29:672, 1960.

Figure 7-19   Modified from West JB: *Ventilation/Blood Flow and Gas Exchange*, ed. 5. Oxford: Blackwell, 1990.

Figure 8-4   From Nielsen M, Smith H: *Acta Physiol Scand* 24:293, 1951.

Figure 8-5   Modified from Loeschke HH, Gertz KH: *Arch Ges Physiol* 267:460, 1958.

Figure 9-3   From Hurtado A: In Dill DB: *Handbook of Physiology, Adaptation to the Environment*. Washington, DC: American Physiological Society, 1964.

Figure 10-6   Modified from Comroe JH: *The Lung: Clinical Physiology and Pulmonary Function Tests*, ed. 2. Chicago, Year Book, 1965.

Subject Index

Page numbers set in *italics* denote figures; those
followed by a "t" denote tables.